# The Practical Management of Asthma

# The Practical Management of Asthma

Editors

**ARTHUR DAWSON, M.D.**

Head, Division of Chest Medicine
Cecil H. and Ida M. Green Hospital
Scripps Clinic and Research Foundation
La Jolla, California


**RONALD A. SIMON, M.D.**

Division of Allergy and Immunology
Scripps Clinic and Research Foundation
La Jolla, California

**Grune & Stratton, Inc.**
*A Subsidiary of Harcourt Brace Jovanovich, Publishers*

Orlando   San Diego
San Francisco   New York   London
Toronto   Montreal   Sydney   Tokyo   São Paulo

**Library of Congress Cataloging in Publication Data**

Main entry under title:
**The Practical management of asthma.**
  Bibliography
  Includes index.
  1. Asthma. I. Dawson, Arthur. II. Simon, Ronald A.
[DNLM: 1. Asthma—Diagnosis. 2. Asthma—
Therapy. WF 553 P895]
RC591.P7 1984        616.2'38        83-12860
ISBN 0-8089-1595-9

**Grune & Stratton, Inc.**
**Orlando, Florida 32887**

Distributed in the United Kingdom by
**Grune & Stratton, Inc. (London) Ltd.**
**24/28 Oval Road, London NW 1**

Library of Congress Catalog Number   83-12860
International Standard Book Number   0-8089-1595-9

Printed in the United States of America

# Contents

# Introduction

From England it is reported that 10% of the patients enrolled in a general practice medical program will at some time require treatment for symptoms of asthma. The number of asthmatics in the United States is estimated at 8.9 million; this number probably represents only a fraction of the patients who have requested medical help because of symptoms due to reversible bronchial obstruction. Fifteen or twenty million might be a closer approximation of the whole asthmatic population if these "occasional asthmatics" are included. Clearly, asthma is one of the most common medical problems encountered by the primary care physician.

This book is based on our experience in teaching the practical management of asthma to practicing physicians. Our program appealed equally to family practitioners, internists, allergists, and chest physicians, and we concluded that there was a real need for a publication covering the practical aspects of managing bronchospastic patients. The number of these patients is so great that most will be seen by primary care physicians and will not be referred to specialists. Judging from the patients we see at Scripps Clinic—who, no doubt, represent a subset of "problem asthmatics"—there must be tens of thousands of Americans who suffer a great deal of unnecessary distress and disability because the nature of their disease is not appreciated or their treatment is not optimal. It is our belief that the great majority of asthmatics can be kept free of symptoms most of the time on a simple and safe outpatient regimen.

In the last few years there have been several important developments in the treatment of asthma. Not only have new therapeutic methods appeared, but better use is being made of some of the older medications such as theophylline and prednisone. Paradoxically, these advances have made it more difficult for the nonspecialist to treat asthma. With the greater number of effective drugs available, more experience and judgment are required to decide what combination to use and when to use it. With the greater range and sophistication of diagnostic tests, it is more difficult to strike an appropriate balance between making a thorough evaluation and squandering the patient's money.

Many exciting discoveries have also been made in the last decade in the fundamental pathophysiology of bronchospasm. If we have little to say about them in this handbook, it is not because we belittle their importance to practicing physicians. We do believe that many publications and teaching programs intended for clinicians tend to give disproportionate emphasis to the biochemical mechanisms of bronchospasm and to deal in a perfunctory way with those details of diagnosis and treatment that are so essential to successful management of the patient. The interested reader will find basic science aspects of asthma well discussed in a number of excellent texts and review articles. This manual brings together a discussion of many details of treatment that may not be found easily in the standard sources. Various aspects of diagnosis and management of asthma are covered in the standard textbook style, and the final section consists of a series of illustrative case reports. These patients' reports were not selected because they represent uncommon or unusually difficult problems, but because they help to flesh out the preceding chapters by showing some of the approaches of physicians who treat asthmatic patients on an everyday basis.

The bulk of this book was written by the staff of Scripps Clinic, but we have been ably assisted by our colleagues in San Diego—Dr. Stephen I. Wasserman of the University of California, and Doctors Michael Schatz and Robert S. Zeiger of the Kaiser Permanente Medical Care Program. For the important and specialized topic of occupational asthma, we have drawn upon the expert knowledge of Dr. Jordan N. Fink of the University of Wisconsin. Our intention in making relatively limited use of outside authorities was to present a coherent approach to the treatment of asthma representing the thinking of a group of specialists working together who often consult on the same patients, and who were able to discuss each others' separate chapters informally as the book went through the months of gestation. By including approximately equal contributions from allergists and chest physicians, we have tried to present a balance between their somewhat different approaches to the management of asthma.

It is our hope that this book will help readers to recognize and treat successfully the majority of their asthmatic patients.

# Contributors

**BRUCE W. ARMSTRONG, JR, Pa-C**
Division of Chest Medicine
Scripps Clinic and Research Foundation
La Jolla, California

**ARTHUR DAWSON, M.D.**
Head, Division of Chest Medicine
Scripps Clinic and Research Foundation
La Jolla, California

**JORDAN N. FINK, M.D.**
Chief, Allergy-Immunology Section
Department of Medicine
Medical College of Wisconsin
Milwaukee, Wisconsin

**WALTER L. JENSEN, M.D.**
Division of Chest Medicine
Scripps Clinic and Research Foundation
La Jolla, California

**LAWRENCE E. KLINE, D.O.**
Division of Chest Medicine
Scripps Clinic and Research Foundation
La Jolla, California

**DIANE LISCHIO, R.N., M.P.H.**
Division of Allergy and Immunology
Scripps Clinic and Research Foundation
La Jolla, California

**DAVID A. MATHISON, M.D.**
Head, Division of Allergy and Immunology
Scripps Clinic and Research Foundation
La Jolla, California

**ALAN H. ROBERTS, Ph.D.**

Director, Behavioral Medicine Program
Scripps Clinic and Research Foundation
La Jolla, California

**ROBERT B. SARNOFF, M.D.**

Division of Chest Medicine
Scripps Clinic and Research Foundation
La Jolla, California

**MICHAEL SCHATZ, M.D.**

Allergy Department
Kaiser Permanente Medical Care Program
San Diego, California

**RONALD A. SIMON, M.D.**

Division of Allergy and Immunology
Scripps Clinic and Research Foundation
La Jolla, California

**DONALD D. STEVENSON, M.D.**

Division of Allergy and Immunology
Scripps Clinic and Research Foundation
La Jolla, California

**STEPHEN I. WASSERMAN, M.D.**

Associate Professor of Medicine
University of California
School of Medicine
University Hospital
San Diego, California

**ROBERT S. ZEIGER, M.D., Ph.D.**

Chief, Department of Allergy and Immunology
Kaiser Permanente Medical Care Program
San Diego, California

# Part 1

# Background

ARTHUR DAWSON
RONALD A. SIMON

**1**

# Bronchospastic Disorders: An Overview

Asthma has been defined as "a disease characterized by an increased responsiveness of the airways to various stimuli and manifested by slowing of forced expiration, which changes in severity either spontaneously or with treatment." In contrast to some earlier definitions, this one, adopted by the American Thoracic Society and the American College of Chest Physicians, makes no reference to the etiology or to immune mechanisms, recognizing that variable obstruction of the airways can occur in response to a number of stimuli.

In addition, this definition of asthma represents a relaxation of older and stricter ideas of the disease in stating only that the obstruction of the airways changes in severity either spontaneously or with treatment. Therefore, we could describe as asthmatic all patients with chronic obstructive lung disease who show a significant variable component to their airways obstruction, even if most of the obstruction is due to permanent anatomical changes. Obviously, it would be very confusing if we used the same diagnosis of asthma to describe the range of patients from children who experience an occasional attack of wheezing to the older people with chronic obstructive pulmonary disease (COPD) who derive some benefit from their bronchodilator inhalers. From the therapeutic point of view however these patients have something in common. Since therapy is the focus of this book, we shall include their various disorders in this chapter on the bronchospastic disorders.

## COMPONENTS OF THE BRONCHOSPASTIC REACTION

The bronchospastic reaction consists not only of bronchial smooth muscle constriction, but also increased bronchial mucus secretion and cough. This combination of reactions, when it occurs in appropriate circumstances, presumably serves the useful function of protecting the lower respiratory tract from aspiration of foreign materials and infectious agents. In the bronchospastic patient, these protective reactions occur in inappropriate circumstances or their intensity and duration are much greater than is necessary for the protective function.

The characteristic feature of asthma, therefore, is abnormally increased responsiveness of the airways to various stimuli. The cause of this hyperreactivity is unknown, but in individual patients it probably represents a mixture of genetic predisposition with humoral, neurogenic, and enivronmental factors interacting in varying degrees. Bronchial hyperreactivity is more than a theoretical concept. Abnormal bronchoconstriction in response to aerosols of histamine or methacholine can be demonstrated not only in those with a history of asthma, but also in many of their asymptomatic relatives.

## MECHANISMS OF BRONCHIAL OBSTRUCTION

In the majority of patients suffering from the bronchospastic disorders, bronchial obstruction results not only from constriction of the bronchial smooth muscle, but also from anatomic changes that cause narrowing of the bronchial lumen. These changes occur in the conducting airways themselves (chronic bronchitis). Airways obstruction can also result from destruction of the lung parenchyma (emphysema). Unfortunately, the terms "chronic bronchitis" and "emphysema" have been used so variously by clinicians, pathologists, and respiratory physiologists that they have become very confusing. Therefore, the expressions "mural obstruction" and "extramural obstruction" will be used here to distinguish two important mechanisms of chronic obstructive disease of the airways.

### Mural Obstruction

This condition results from several different processes that can combine to cause narrowing of the bronchial lumen. These include mucosal edema, thickening of the mucosa and submucosa resulting from mucus gland hypertrophy and inflammatory cell infiltration, hypertrophy of the bronchial muscle layers, and postinflammatory fibrosis of the bronchial and peribronchial tissues. Some of these pathologic changes are at least potentially reversible, but eventually there is more or less permanent anatomic change in the bronchial wall.

### Extramural Obstruction

In extramural obstruction there is bronchial narrowing through destruction of the elastic elements in the lung parenchyma that normally maintain the patency of the collapsible intrathoracic airways. The recoil pressure of the lung exerts an outward force from the lumen at each point of attachment of the parenchymal structures. As the elastic elements are destroyed, the recoil force diminishes and the airways tend to collapse.

The smaller the airways and the thinner their walls, the more they depend on the recoil pressure of the lung to maintain their normal patency (Fig. 1-1). Therefore, the principal site of extramural obstruction (emphysema) is the terminal airways. Bronchoconstriction, by contrast, is most prominent in larger airways that are abundantly supplied with smooth muscle. Mural obstruction due to various mechanisms probably can affect conducting airways of all sizes down to the terminal level. Presumably this accounts for the rather disappointing results of trying to classify patients as having large airways or small airways obstruction in order to predict their response to treatment. However, the concept of mural and extramural obstruction is helpful as an aid to understanding the interplay between potentially treatable and nontreatable components in chronic airways obstruction.

### Mucus Plugging

When bronchial obstruction has persisted for a period of hours or days, there is a tendency for secretions to accumulate in the lumen. With severe bronchospasm, the secretions become more viscous as the cough becomes less effective as a result of fatigue, dehydration, and certain medications. In extreme cases, "bronchial casts" may form,

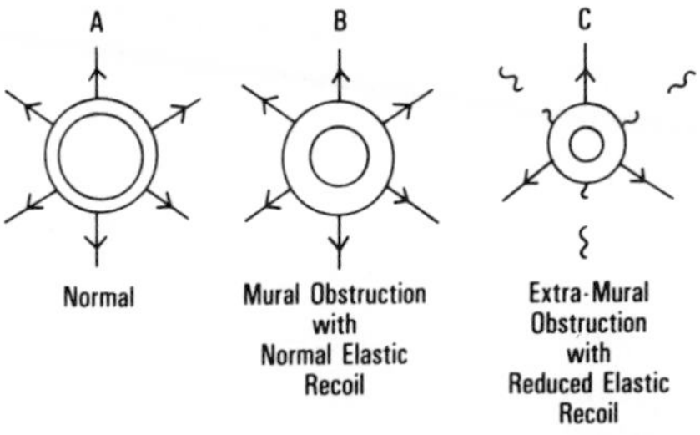

**Fig. 1-1.**   Mural Obstruction Diagram. Normal; Mural obstruction with normal elastic recoil; Extra-mural obstruction with
reduced elastic recoil.

extending to occlude segmental, lobar, and even mainstem bronchi, and at this stage the
usual pharmacologic agents are ineffective even if they can increase the size of the lumen.
When mucus plugging reaches this degree, the diagnosis "mucus impaction syndrome"
becomes appropriate, but lesser degrees of mucus impaction probably are important in
delaying recovery from many episodes of acute bronchospasm.

## BRONCHOSPASTIC COPD

The chest physician sees relatively few patients with simple spasmodic or episodic
asthma. Most older patients suffering from the bronchospastic disorders have chronic and
nonreversible airways obstruction with more or less of a superimposed bronchospastic
component. It is essential to recognize this reversible element of their disease because even
a small improvement in their bronchial obstruction can have a major beneficial effect on
their life-style. It is important to include discussion of bronchospastic COPD in this book
because these patients respond to the same medications and other therapeutic interventions
that are used so successfully in uncomplicated asthma. Often they have been inappropriately told by friends, or even unfortunately by a physician, that they have emphysema
and that "nothing can be done for it." It is a great help in approaching these patients to tell
them that they have "a form of asthma"—and, as explained earlier, they certainly do have
a form of asthma according to the currently accepted definition. Treatment of such patients
can be a very gratifying experience because the modest reversal of the airways obstruction
that can be achieved may seem almost miraculous to them, especially if they have had
severely obstructed airways for years.

## A PHYSIOLOGIC CLASSIFICATION OF THE
## BRONCHOSPASTIC DISORDERS

Probably any person would develop bronchospasm in response to a sufficiently
intense stimulus. Bronchoconstriction can be triggered in an asthmatic by stimuli that do
not cause this reaction in most normal individuals, however. The bronchospastic disorders
can be classified according to the nature of the stimulus, an etiologic classification, or
according to the disturbance of function of the airways, a physiologic classification.

*Bronchial hyperreactivity.*  Increased responsiveness of the airways to a variety of stimuli is a characteristic and perhaps invariable feature of the bronchospastic disorders. Here the term is used to refer to that large reservoir of potential asthmatics who have no bronchial obstruction at the time of testing and who sometimes give no history of asthma. They can be identified only by an abnormal response to inhalation challenge testing with drugs such as histamine or methacholine.[1] It is believed that this population of potential asthmatics is a reservoir of adult-onset clinical asthma cases. Until long-term follow-up studies have been done on otherwise normal subjects with bronchial hyperreactivity, however, this is only speculation.

*Acute episodic asthma.*  This term has been used for those patients who experience attacks of bronchospasm but whose lung function is normal, or nearly so, between attacks.

*Chronic asthmatic bronchitis.*  In these patients bronchospasm is perennial, although it is periodically exacerbated with acute attacks.

*Chronic obstructive lung disease with bronchospasm.*  This type of disease has already been mentioned (bronchospastic COPD). In many of these cases there will be no reported history of attacks of wheezing or exacerbations of dyspnea except, perhaps, at the time of an acute respiratory infection. These patients are recognized by their response to bronchodilator therapy. These patients constitute a large and important group, especially to the chest physician and the primary care internist.

## NONBRONCHOSPASTIC CAUSES OF WHEEZING

The following list includes a wide variety of disorders that should be ruled out whenever a diagnosis of asthma is suspected but especially when the case and setting appear atypical or the response to treatment is poor:[2]

1. Congestive heart failure
2. Pulmonary embolism
3. Increased airway collapsability (tracheomalacia and bronchomalacia)
4. Chronic bronchitis with mucosal edema and secretions
5. Endobronchial disease: tumor, foreign body, granulomatous inflammation
6. External bronchial compression
7. Substernal thyroid

## ETIOLOGIC CLASSIFICATION (PROVOKING FACTORS)

In 1918 Rackemann[3] recognized that not all asthma was caused by allergy to inhalants or ingestants (extrinsic), and he used the term "intrinsic asthma" for those cases where "the cause lies within the patient's body." In the years since Rackemann's report, this classification has proved useful and has gained widespread acceptance. However, there is so much heterogeneity among asthmatic patients that it is no longer sufficient to consider them simply as "extrinsic," "intrinsic," or "mixed." We believe that successful management of the asthmatic patient depends on a systematic search for potential

Table 1-1
**Provoking Factors in Bronchial Asthma: 1-Year Prospective Study of 234 Patients**

| Provoking Factor | Patients with Factor (%) | | |
| --- | --- | --- | --- |
| | Sole | Major | Contributing |
| Immediate hypersensitivity infection | 5.1 | 25 | 45 |
| Acute upper respiratory illness | 2.6 | 7 | 19 |
| Sinusitis | 1.3 | 9 | 23 |
| Acute bronchitis (purulent sputum) | 1.3 | 3 | 12 |
| Postviral onset | 0.4 | 7 | 11 |
| Aspirin intolerance | 0.9 | 9 | 10 |
| Asthmatic bronchitis (COPD) | 0.9 | 17 | 20 |
| Isoproterenol abuse | 0.0 | 0.4 | 4 |
| Irritant inhalation | 0.0 | 3 | 24 |
| Exercise | 0.0 | 0.4 | 18 |
| Atmospheric change | 0.0 | 0.4 | 21 |
| Emotional upset | 0.0 | 1.7 | 9.8 |
| Associated disease | 0.0 | 0.4 | 1.7 |
| Idiopathic | 10.0 | | |
| Total | 22.5 | 83.3 | |

mechanisms and settings that may aggravate the asthmatic state. Provoking factors in bronchial asthma that we look for are listed in Table 1-1.[4]

## Allergies

In a prospective study of 234 adult patients presenting to the Allergy and Immunology Division at Scripps Clinic in the early 1970s, only 58 (25%) had asthma in which an allergic immunoglobulin E (IgE)-mediated immediate hypersensitivity mechanism was the major provoking factor. In an additional 47 patients, allergic mechanisms were judged to be minor provoking factors. Even with these two groups combined, only 45% of the patients had "allergic" asthma. Other studies have shown the frequency of allergic asthma to vary from 56% to 66%, depending on the patients' age (with an increased incidence in children), the population studied, and the criteria used to establish the diagnosis. In the Scripps Clinic study, to incriminate immediate hypersensitivity as contributing to the asthmatic state, we required documentation of skin-sensitizing antibodies (reagins) to allergens to which the patient is exposed, and evidence from the history or—even better—controlled inhalation challenges that these allergens indeed provoke asthmatic symptoms.[5] Although 66% of patients had positive wheal and flare skin tests to one or more antigen tested, 31 of the 234 had positive skin tests only to allergens not present in their environment.

Only about one-third of the patients who were challenged with inhaled extracts of the allergens to which they had shown positive skin tests developed a bronchospastic response. Therefore, when the 31 patients with irrelevant but positive skin test were combined with the 18 patients who had negative bronchial challenges to relevant positive skin tests, there was a total of 49 patients with reaginic antibodies that were not contributing to their asthma.

It has been well documented that positive skin tests can be found in up to 20% to 25% of the general population, most of them individuals with no previous respiratory complaints.[6-9] From these studies, we feel strongly that the mere presence of reaginic antibodies does not establish that they are causally related to the asthma.

## Infection

It is noteworthy that infections (sinusitis, upper respiratory infections, acute bronchitis, and postviral reactions) were the most common major provoking factor in the Scripps study. Although the majority of patients in this study had abnormal sinus roentgenograms, only occasionally were we able to culture bacteria from the affected sinus.[10] Therefore, it is believed that only air fluid levels or total opacification of sinuses warrant specific therapy or additional workup. In patients with flares of asthma coinciding with upper respiratory infections or purulent sputum, we rarely were able to culture pathogenic bacteria from the transtracheal secretions.[11] This suggests that most "infectious" exacerbations of bronchospasm are caused by viral infections[12] or by noninfectious provoking factors. There is evidence that in children many asthmatic relapses are triggered by rhinoviruses.

## Irritants

Inhaled irritants include tobacco smoke, air pollution, and dusts that do not produce an IgE-mediated reaction. There has been no demonstration of IgE antibodies directed against tobacco in either smoke-sensitive or non–smoke-sensitive individuals.[13] Although dust is capable of inducing an IgE response in certain atopic individuals, it can clearly provoke asthma relapses due purely to the irritation from inhalation of dust particles. The role of air pollution in bronchial asthma is complex and difficult to evaluate. There are conflicting reports correlating asthma activity and air pollution levels for groups of patients, but individual patients commonly complain that air pollution, especially smog, exacerbates their asthma. It is quite clear, from experimental studies, that asthmatics are significantly more sensitive to sulfur dioxide, especially during exercise.[14] There is further discussion of asthma and the home environment in Chapter 18.

## Thyroid Disease and Asthma

Bronchial asthma has been associated with both hypothyroidism and hyperthyroid-ism.[15-17] A number of studies in the literature have revealed that hyperthyroidism increases the severity of bronchial asthma. There is less evidence that hypothyroidism affects asthma, although some anecdotal reports have suggested that asthma may improve with the development of thyroid deficiency.

There are a number of theories that relate to this, but none of them has been substantiated. One explanation is based on the interactions of thyroid hormones and cyclic adenosine monophosphate (cAMP). The excessive breakdown of adenosine triphosphate (ATP) in hyperthyroidism would decrease the levels of (cAMP) and so increase asthma activity. It has also been shown that excessive thyroid hormone increases the degradation of hydrocortisone to its inactive 11-keto metabolites.

Over the years, we have seen several patients with complaints of periodic shortness of breath, dyspnea, and sometimes dizziness and chest pain. These patients had been referred to us for evaluation and treatment of bronchial asthma although there was no history of wheezing, chest congestion, or cough. Laboratory studies confirmed the diagnosis of hyperthyroidism, and pulmonary function tests showed no evidence of reversible airways disease.

Any asthmatic who is to be on long-term iodide therapy should be observed carefully for iodide-induced changes in thyroid function. Hypothyroidism commonly develops during long-term administration of expectorants and bronchodilator mixtures containing iodides. There are also reports of exacerbation of bronchial asthma when thyroid function returns after administration of an iodine-containing expectorant is discontinued. A much less common condition is iodine-induced thyrotoxicosis (the Jod-Basedow phenomenon). However, there are several isolated case reports of bronchial asthma aggravated by iodine-induced hyperthyroidism.[18]

## Other Provoking Factors

Our group at Scripps Clinic has been especially interested in aspirin sensitivity and asthma.[19,20] There has also been much recent investigation of the asthma provoked by cold air and by exercise.[21]

The other major provoking factors are listed in Table 1-1. Even if one contributing factor seems to be predominant, the physician should not neglect to search for others, especially in a patient who is not doing well. Chronic sinusitis, abuse of inhaled sympathomimetics, or emotional factors may easily pass undetected.

In reviewing the list of provoking factors, one is struck by the heterogenous and complex pattern of interactions that can trigger an asthmatic attack. Such a pattern is consistent with the underlying immunologic, physiologic, and biochemical factors that influence the bronchial muscles and mucous membranes.

## REFERENCES

1.  Parker CD, Bilbo RE, Reed CE: Methacholine aerosol as test for bronchial asthma. Arch Intern Med 115:452, 1965
2.  Moser KM: Wheezing during forced expiration: Differential diagnosis. JAMA 244:1852, 1980
3.  Rackemann FM: A clinical study of 150 cases of bronchial asthma. Arch Intern Med 22:517, 1918
4.  Stevenson DD, Mathison DA, Tan EM, et al: Provoking factors in bronchial asthma. Arch Intern Med 135:777, 1975
5.  Popa V, Teceluscu D, Stanescu D, et al: The value of inhalation tests in perennial bronchial asthma. J Allergy Clin Immunol 42:130, 1968
6.  Buffum WP: Diagnosis of asthma in infancy. J Ped 52:264, 1968
7.  Hill LW: Certain aspects of allergy in children: A critical review of recent literature. N Engl J Med 265:1248, 1961
8.  Barbee RA, Lebowitz MD, Thompson HC, et al: Immediate skin test reactivity in a general population sample. Intern Med 84:129, 1976
9.  Curran WS, Goldman G: The incidence of immediately reacting allergy skin tests in a "normal" adult population. J Allergy 32:392, 1961
10. Berman SZ, Mathison DA, Stevenson DD, et al: Maxillary sinusitis in bronchial asthma. J Allergy Clin Immunol 53:311, 1974

11. Berman SZ, Mathison DA, Stevenson DD, et al: Transtracheal aspiration studies in asthmatic patients in relapse with "infective" asthma and in subjects without respiratory disease. J Allergy Clin Immunol 56:206, 1975

12. Miner TC, Dick EC, DeMeo AN, et al: Viruses as precipitants of asthmatic attacks in children. JAMA 227:298, 1974

13. Lehrer SD, Wilson MR, Karr RM, et al: IgE antibody response of smokers, nonsmokers, and "smoke sensitive" persons to tobacco leaf and smoke antigens. Am Rev Respir Dis 121:168, 1980

14. Sheppard D, Saisho A, Nadel JA, et al: Exercise increases sulfur dioxide induced bronchoconstriction in asthmatic subjects. Am Rev Respir Dis 123:486–491, 1981

15. Bush RK, Ehrlich EN, Reed CE: Thyroid disease in asthma. J Allergy Clin Immunol 59:398, 1977

16. Settipane GA, Schoenfeld E, Hamolsky NW: Asthma and hyperthyroidism. J Allergy Clin Immunol 49:348, 1972

17. Corsager S, Ostergaard-Kristensen HP: Iodine induced hypothyroidism and its effect on the severity of asthma. Acta Med Scand 205:115, 1979

18. Gutknetch DR: Asthma complicated by iodine-induced thyrotoxicosis (letter). New Engl J Med 256:236, 1977

19. Stevenson DD, Simon RA, Mathison DA: Aspirin sensitive asthma: Tolerance to aspirin after positive oral aspirin challenge. J Allergy Clin Immunol 66:82–88, 1980

20. Pleskow WW, Stevenson DD, Mathison DA, et al: Aspirin desensitization in aspirin sensitive asthmatic patients: Clinical manifestations and characterization of the refractory period. J Allergy Clin Immunol 69:11–19, 1982

21. McFadden ER Jr, Ingram RH Jr: Exercise induced asthma: Observations on the initiating stimulus. New Engl J Med 301:763–769, 1979

# PART 2

# Approach to the Bronchospastic Patient

# 2

DAVID A. MATHISON

# History Taking: Search for Environmental and Other Aggravating Factors

To manage the asthmatic patient, the practitioner needs to identify those factors that initiate, aggravate, or perpetuate the asthmatic attack.[1] Some of the currently recognized factors, the setting in which they operate, and the diagnostic tests relevant to them, as well as some recommendations for treatment, are listed in Table 2-1. The patient's history provides the best clues as to the importance of various aggravating factors. A single factor rarely accounts for all asthma attacks.

## IMMEDIATE HYPERSENSITIVITY

Asthma attributed to immediate hypersensitivity (IgE-mediated) reaction is also called "allergic" or "extrinsic" asthma.[2] This form of asthma ordinarily appears first in childhood; is associated with hay fever, or acute pruritic rhinoconjunctivitis due to IgE reaction to aeroallergen; and consistently is exacerbated by exposures to the aeroallergens to which the individual is sensitive. In taking the history, the practicioner seeks to link exacerbations to exposures to aeroallergens. The key questions for IgE-mediated asthma relate to whether the attacks are seasonal, perennial, or sporadic; whether the asthma is related to occupation; and what is in the air that might account for the reaction.[3]

*Seasonal* occurrence of hay feaver-asthma suggests IgE-mediated reaction to pollens or mold spores. In general, trees pollenate in early spring, grasses in late spring and early summer, and weeds in late summer to frost. The grass-sensitive patient usually has an exacerbation of symptoms while mowing the lawn. Airborne spores are generated from fungi that grow in microscopic colonies in moist and decaying vegetation. Outdoor spore counts are greatest during rainy periods and in the fall until snow covers the ground. The allergist knowledgeable about the aerobiology in the particular geographic area can often, by history alone, pinpoint the responsible tree, grass pollen, ragweed, or *Alternaria* spore by correlating the severity of symptoms with the pollen and spore counts.

*Perennial* rhinitis-asthma, which is exacerbated by late fall and winter conditions, suggests IgE sensitivity to aeroallergens within the home. House dust and mites, animal proteins, and fungal spores are the inhaled substances within the home most likely to provoke IgE-triggered asthma.

House dust usually contains fibrous materials of plant and synthetic origin, human epidermis, fungi, bacteria, food remnants, inorganic substances, mites, and—in some

**Table 2-1**

**Initiating, Aggravating, and Perpetuating Factors in Asthma**

| Mechanism–Association | Setting | Diagnostic Studies | Treatment |
|---|---|---|---|
| Immediate hypersensitivity (IgE-mediated allergic or extrinsic) | Exposure to inhalant allergen precipitates asthmatic episode, frequently associated with rhinoconjunctivitis | History; Wheal-flare skin tests; Inhalation challenge | Avoidance of allergens; Hyposensitization; Symptomatic |
| Aeroirritant | Smoke or other irritant exposure | History | Avoidance; Symptomatic |
| Respiratory infection Acute viral | Relapse of asthma coincides with or follows head cold | Nose and pharynx examination; viral serology | Symptomatic |
| Bacterial bronchitis or sinusitis | Relapse of asthma coincides with or follows change of sputum production or color | Sputum and nose cultures; Sinus x-rays | Antimicrobial; Symptomatic |
| Postviral onset | Flulike syndrome evolves into persistent cough, then asthma | Viral serology | Symptomatic |
| Exercise—cooling and drying of airway | During or following vigorous exercise | Treadmill exercise provocation | Preexercise bronchodilator or cromolyn |
| Meteorologic changes | Temperature, humidity, or barometric pressure change | History | Symptomatic |
| Emotional | Emotional upset–laughter, anger preceeds relapse of asthma | History | Symptomatic |
| Inhaler abuse | Increased use of sympathomimetic cartridge nebulizer with decreased symptom relief | Spirometry before, 5, and 60 minutes after inhaler use | Discontinue inhaler |

| | | | |
|---|---|---|---|
| Aspirin sensitivity | Severe asthmatic episode follows ingestion of aspirin; Frequently associated nasal polyps and sinusitis | History | Avoidance of aspirin; Corticosteroids |
| Metabisulfite sensitivity | Asthma during or following restaurant meal | History; Challenge | Avoidance |
| Associated Disease Chronic bronchitis and/or emphysema | History of tobacco smoking | Pulmonary function (irreversible airways obstruction, loss of elastic recoil) | As indicated |
| Sinusitis | Obstruction of sinus drainage by inflammation or infection | History; Sinus transillumination; Sinus x-ray; Culture of aspirate | Drainage; Toilet; Antimicrobial |
| Carcinoid tumor | Bronchial or systemic release of serotonin | Urinary 5-hydroxyindoleacetic acid | Surgery; Symptomatic |
| Esophageal dysfunction | Acid reflux–refex | As indicated | As indicated |
| Cardiac disease (Cardiac asthma) | Cardiac failure | As indicated | As indicated |
| Psychological disorder | High panic or fear potential; Psychiatric disorder; Chronic asthma | MMPI | Behavior modification; Psychotropic drugs; Psychotherapy |
| Bronchopulmonary aspergillosis | Aspergillus colonization of bronchial tree in atopic asthmatic | Wheal-flare skin test; Serum precipitin; Elevated serum IgE; X-ray pulmonary; Infiltrates–central bronchieltasis | Corticosteroid; Toilet |
| Bronchial obstruction | Localized bronchial obstruction (Foreign body, neoplasm) | Bronchoscopy | Surgery |
| Pulmonary embolus | Venous stasis or thrombosis | As indicated | As indicated |

households—proteins from domestic pets and cockroach or other insect parts. Within the past two decades, mites of the genus *Dermatophagoides* (*D. farinae* in the United States) have been shown to be a major allergen in house dust. The allergen is concentrated in fecal particles that are 10–40 $\mu$m in diameter. Dust from the bed and bedroom floor ordinarily contains the highest concentrations of mite allergen.[4] Live mite populations tend to be greatest during warm and humid months, but concentrations of airborne mite antigen increase during colder months when forced-air heating systems are operating. This increase of circulating mite allergen may account for late fall and winter exacerbations of asthma.

Household pets, including cats, dogs, and rodents, disseminate aeroallergens in the form of proteins desquamated from the epidermis or excreted in saliva or urine. Individual hypersensitivity to these proteins may be so exquisite that even brief exposures to households occupied by animals may precipitate severe asthma. Avian proteins originating from feather pillows or down comforters may also trigger asthmatic attacks in the hypersensitive individual.

Airborne spores are generated from fungi that grow in moist areas of the home, including food storage areas, garbage containers, soiled upholstery, carpets, rubber and synthetic foams, and soil and drainage pans of overwatered house plants. Poorly maintained cold-mist vaporizers and console humdifiers may emit dense fungus aerosols. Damage from breaks in waterlines or flooding of carpets and floors produces an evironment highly conducive to fungal proliferation. Small-spored species of *Penicillium* and *Aspergillus, Rizopus,* and *Mucor* as well as unicellular yeasts ordinarily dominate the microflora within the household.

*Sporadic* episodes of acute rhinoconjunctivitis with asthma are often recognized by the patient as an allergic reaction to cat, dog, or house dust. When an IgE reaction to ingested food excerbates asthma, there usually is accompanying gastrointestinal distress or urticaria. In contrast to the evaluation of urticaria, the dietary history is only occasionally relevant to asthma.

Occupational environmental exposures that trigger IgE-mediated asthma are reviewed in Chapters 18 and 24 of this volume.

Patients with allergic or extrinsic asthma tend to have a family history of one of the atopic disorders, hay fever, asthma, or eczema associated with reaginic (IgE) antibodies. Fifty-percent of the children of two mildly atopic parents, will be similarly affected, 25% severely affected, and 25% spared—a pattern of inheritance suggesting codominant expression. All the atopic disorders have their strongest expression in childhood, although persistence throughout adult life is not unusual. Relapse or appearance of asthma in middle or late adulthood in an individual with personal or family history of atopy should not automatically be attributed to IgE mechanisms. So-called intrinsic adult-onset asthma probably occurs more commonly in individuals with a history of atopy than in others.

## OTHER FACTORS IN ASTHMA

The taking of a history for the remaining factors listed in Table 2-1 requires compulsion to prevent omission. Salient features of several factors follow:

### Aeroirritants

These agents aggravate asthma in patients of all ages. Indeed, hyperreactivity of the trachobronchial tree to irritant stimuli is almost always demonstrated in asthma. Perhaps the greatest threat to asthmatic patients is tobacco smoke, so much so that many patients consider themselves "allergic" to smoke despite the fact that IgE reactivity to smoke per se does not account for the reaction.[5] Other aeroirritants in the home may include fumes from cooking and heating appliances, dusts and fumes from chemical cleaners (especially oven cleaning) and gardening aids, fresh newsprint, smoke from fireplaces, aromatic terpenes from evergreen Christmas trees, and aerosols from hair sprays and other "helpful" products. Asthma is among the disorders that have been noted by occupants of homes insulated with urea formaldehyde foam and mobile homes constructed with formaldehyde-treated plywood or particle board.[6] Outdoor air pollutants, particularly photochemical smog, contribute to exacerbations of asthma.[7]

### Respiratory Infection

The viruses that cause the common cold or tracheobronchitis often trigger an asthmatic attack. These viruses vary in their propensity to produce asthmatic relapse, but respiratory syncytial and influenza viruses frequently trigger a severe exacerbation. The appearance of congestion, pain, or tenderness localized to one or several of the paranasal sinuses and accompanied by discolored purulent discharge from the nose or nasopharynx suggests acute bacterial sinusitis; cough with production of discolored or purulent sputum suggests acute bacterial bronchitis. *Haemophilus influenzae* and *Streptococcus pneumoniae* are the bacteria most likely to produce acute sinusitis[8] and bronchitis. Late-adult-onset asthma (also referred to as "intrinsic" asthma) sometimes evolves following influenza or other viral illness, with months of persistent cough followed by attacks of dyspnea and wheezing.

### Exercise Induced Asthma

Exercise-induced asthma is typified by bronchoconstriction that occurs about 5 minutes into vigorous exercise, peaks 5–10 minutes after cessation of exercise, and remits spontaneously over 30–90 minutes.[9] The degree of airway obstruction that develops for any given exercise task is an inverse function of the inspired-air temperature and humidity; the colder and drier the air, the greater the bronchoconstrictive response. Thus swimming is the least asthmagenic exercise.

### Emotional Upset

Activities that alter breathing, such as vigorous laughter or shouting, will precipitate bronchoconstriction, especially in the asthmatic individual already in mild relapse. The role of psychological factors and psychiatric disorders in asthma are listed in Table 2-1 as "associated disease" and are further discussed in Chapter 20.

### Inhaler Abuse

Abuse of inhalers that compounds and perpetuates asthmatic relapse was initially recognized in patients who overused isoproterenol delivered from pressurized cartridge nebulizers.[10] The more selective beta agonists (See Chapter 9), especially those with a long duration of action (e.g., albuterol) are less likely to be overused. Nonetheless, if the patient admits to using a cartridge nebulizer more often than once an hour or consuming a cartridge in less than a fortnight, inhaler abuse should be suspected.

### Aspirin Sensitivity

Aspirin sensitivity[11] in asthmatic patients is characterized by acute flush, rhinorrhea, and severe asthmatic attack within an hour or so of ingesting ordinary doses of aspirin or an aspirinlike drug (see Chapter 7). The majority of aspirin-sensitive asthmatic patients also have chronic rhinosinusitis with nasal polyps. Approximately 35% of patients with the combination of rhinosinusitis, nasal polyps, and intrinsic asthma and 8% of all asthmatic patients are sensitive to aspirin. The mechanisms underlying the respiratory responses to aspirin are not understood. There is no evidence of an IgE-mediated reaction. Sensitivity to tartazine [Food and Drug Administration (FDA) Yellow Dye No. 5] has been reported in a very small minority of aspirin-sensitive asthmatic patients.

### Sulfite

Sulfite sensitivity has been recognized in several asthmatic patients[12] who experienced sudden asthmatic relapse while ingesting foods and drinks in restaurants. Metabisulfite and other sulfites are used as preservatives and antioxidants; they are sprayed on fresh fruits and vegetables, and shellfish, or added to beer, and wine. Sensitivity to these preservatives may be as common as aspirin sensitivity.

### Chronic Sinusitis

Chronic sinusitis, as demonstrated by roentgenographic abnormality of the sinuses, is found in the majority of asthmatic patients.[13] Mucoid or mucopurulent drainage from the upper respiratory tract into the tracheobronchial tree can perpetuate the asthma problem.

### Esophageal Dysfunction

Esophageal dysfunction, espeically gastroesophageal reflux with reflex bronchospasm, is not uncommon in overweight adult asthmatic patients and may be compounded by theophylline therapy, which tends to reduce the lower esophageal sphincter pressure. Treatment of the reflux also improves respiratory symptoms in afflicted patients.[14]

### Bronchopulmonary Aspergillosis

Bronchopulmonary aspergillosis is a syndrome of asthma[15] complicated by recurrent pulmonary infiltrates and central bronchiectasis due to immunologic reactions to *Aspergillus fumigatus* (or other aspergillus species) colonizing the bronchial tree. The diagnosis is likely if wheal-flare cutaneous reactivity and serum precipitins to aspergillus can be demonstrated and if the serum IgE concentration is elevated above 2000 IU/ml (see Chapter 5).

In summary, history-taking from the asthmatic patient offers an opportunity to identify environmental and other factors that cause exacerbations and influence the course of the disease. A systematic approach, including a search for each of the factors listed in Table 2-1, may be helpful in the management of the individual patient. Appended is a questionnaire that we use at Scripps Clinic to facilitate the physician's history-taking for asthma and other allergic disorders.

SCRIPPS CLINIC MEDICAL GROUP, INC.
Allergy · Immunology Review

Name _____ Date _____

Occupation _____

PLEASE NOTE:

Antihistamine medications (Benadryl, Atarax, Contac, etc.) may interfere with skin tests for specific allergies; if possible, we would prefer that you stop antihistamine medications 48 hours before your evaluation in the ALLERGY and IMMUNOLOGY DIVISION. You need not stop other medications.

Please answer all questions on all four pages to the best of your ability. Base your answers on your own observations and not on what you have been told by others or what you may have presumed on the basis of previous allergy tests. Complete the questionnaire before you see the doctor as the information will organize your thinking and facilitate understanding of your case.

I. Describe in your own words the problem(s) you are having which you think might be on the basis of

an allergic (exaggerated) reaction: _____

_____

_____

_____

_____

_____

II. Check the boxes which apply to your symptoms:

| | Present Problem | Past Problem | Physician Comment |
|---|---|---|---|
| A. Eye symptoms: | | | |
| Itching | ☐ | ☐ | |
| Watering | ☐ | ☐ | |
| Redness | ☐ | ☐ | |
| Swelling | ☐ | ☐ | |
| Burning | ☐ | ☐ | |
| Dryness | ☐ | ☐ | |
| B. Symptoms in the upper respiratory tract (nose, sinuses, throat, eustachian tubes, voice box)? | | | |
| Itching | ☐ | ☐ | |
| Sneezing | ☐ | ☐ | |
| Congestion | ☐ | ☐ | |
| Headache | ☐ | ☐ | |
| Obstruction | ☐ | ☐ | |
| Drainage | ☐ | ☐ | |
| Soreness | ☐ | ☐ | |
| Dryness | ☐ | ☐ | |
| Hoarseness | ☐ | ☐ | |
| Hearing loss | ☐ | ☐ | |
| Polyps | ☐ | ☐ | |
| Loss of Smell/Taste | ☐ | ☐ | |

345MR780

20

Allergy Immunology Review

| | | Present Problem | Past Problem | Physician Comment |
|---|---|---|---|---|
| C | Symptoms in the lower respiratory tract (windpipe, bronchi, lungs): | | | |
| | Itching | ☐ | ☐ | |
| | Coughing | ☐ | ☐ | |
| | Sputum production | ☐ | ☐ | |
| | Tightness-Congestion | ☐ | ☐ | |
| | Wheezing | ☐ | ☐ | |
| | Shortness of breath | ☐ | ☐ | |
| | Chest soreness | ☐ | ☐ | |
| | Other (Describe) _____ | ☐ | ☐ | |
| D | Symptoms in the stomach and digestive system which you suspect might be allergic: | | | |
| | Pain or difficulty swallowing | ☐ | ☐ | |
| | Nausea or vomiting | ☐ | ☐ | |
| | Abdominal cramping | ☐ | ☐ | |
| | Diarrhea | ☐ | ☐ | |
| | Constipation | ☐ | ☐ | |
| | Other (Describe) _____ | ☐ | ☐ | |
| E | Hives or giant swelling? | ☐ | ☐ | |
| F | Eczema? | ☐ | ☐ | |
| G | Skin reaction to poison ivy/oak, metals, chemical or cosmetics? (Circle) | ☐ | ☐ | |
| H | Reaction to bee, hornet, wasp, yellow jacket bit or other stinging insect bite? (Circle) | ☐ | ☐ | |
| I | Reaction to Immunization? | ☐ | ☐ | |
| J | Reaction to drug? | ☐ | ☐ | |
| | Penicillin | ☐ | ☐ | |
| | Aspirin | ☐ | ☐ | |
| | Sulfa | ☐ | ☐ | |
| | Nose drops/sprays | ☐ | ☐ | |
| | Sedatives | ☐ | ☐ | |
| | Pain relievers | ☐ | ☐ | |
| | Hormones | ☐ | ☐ | |
| | Antihistamines | ☐ | ☐ | |
| | Cortisone | ☐ | ☐ | |
| | X-Ray dye | ☐ | ☐ | |
| | Immunization | ☐ | ☐ | |
| | Other _____ | ☐ | ☐ | |

| III. Family History of Allergy | Eyes | Nose/Sinuses | Chest | Digestive | Hives/Swelling | Eczema |
|---|---|---|---|---|---|---|
| Mother | ☐ | ☐ | ☐ | ☐ | ☐ | ☐ |
| Father | ☐ | ☐ | ☐ | ☐ | ☐ | ☐ |
| Siblings | ☐ | ☐ | ☐ | ☐ | ☐ | ☐ |
| Children | ☐ | ☐ | ☐ | ☐ | ☐ | ☐ |

Allergy Immunology Review

IV. Check appropriate box for symptoms aggravated or precipitated by exposure or during:

| | Eyes | Nose/Sinuses/Ears | Chest | Digestive | Hives/Swelling | Eczema |
|---|---|---|---|---|---|---|
| Spring (March-April-May) | ☐ | ☐ | ☐ | ☐ | ☐ | ☐ |
| Summer(June-July-August) | ☐ | ☐ | ☐ | ☐ | ☐ | ☐ |
| Autumn (Sept-Oct-Nov) | ☐ | ☐ | ☐ | ☐ | ☐ | ☐ |
| Winter(Dec-Jan-Feb) | ☐ | ☐ | ☐ | ☐ | ☐ | ☐ |
| Sleep | ☐ | ☐ | ☐ | ☐ | ☐ | ☐ |
| On awakening | ☐ | ☐ | ☐ | ☐ | ☐ | ☐ |
| At work | ☐ | ☐ | ☐ | ☐ | ☐ | ☐ |
| At play | ☐ | ☐ | ☐ | ☐ | ☐ | ☐ |
| Vacation | ☐ | ☐ | ☐ | ☐ | ☐ | ☐ |
| Exercise | ☐ | ☐ | ☐ | ☐ | ☐ | ☐ |
| Emotional Upset | ☐ | ☐ | ☐ | ☐ | ☐ | ☐ |
| Weather changes | ☐ | ☐ | ☐ | ☐ | ☐ | ☐ |
| Dampness | ☐ | ☐ | ☐ | ☐ | ☐ | ☐ |
| Heat | ☐ | ☐ | ☐ | ☐ | ☐ | ☐ |
| Cold | ☐ | ☐ | ☐ | ☐ | ☐ | ☐ |
| Air Conditioning | ☐ | ☐ | ☐ | ☐ | ☐ | ☐ |
| Sunlight | ☐ | ☐ | ☐ | ☐ | ☐ | ☐ |
| Irritant fumes/aerosols/sprays | ☐ | ☐ | ☐ | ☐ | ☐ | ☐ |
| Smog | ☐ | ☐ | ☐ | ☐ | ☐ | ☐ |
| Cosmetics/perfumes | ☐ | ☐ | ☐ | ☐ | ☐ | ☐ |
| Poison ivy/oak | ☐ | ☐ | ☐ | ☐ | ☐ | ☐ |
| Clothing _____ | ☐ | ☐ | ☐ | ☐ | ☐ | ☐ |
| Tobacco smoke | ☐ | ☐ | ☐ | ☐ | ☐ | ☐ |
| Newsprint | ☐ | ☐ | ☐ | ☐ | ☐ | ☐ |
| House dust | ☐ | ☐ | ☐ | ☐ | ☐ | ☐ |
| Road dust | ☐ | ☐ | ☐ | ☐ | ☐ | ☐ |
| Cats | ☐ | ☐ | ☐ | ☐ | ☐ | ☐ |
| Dogs | ☐ | ☐ | ☐ | ☐ | ☐ | ☐ |
| Birds/feathers | ☐ | ☐ | ☐ | ☐ | ☐ | ☐ |
| Horses | ☐ | ☐ | ☐ | ☐ | ☐ | ☐ |
| Other animal(s)_____ | ☐ | ☐ | ☐ | ☐ | ☐ | ☐ |
| Egg | ☐ | ☐ | ☐ | ☐ | ☐ | ☐ |
| Milk/Dairy Products | ☐ | ☐ | ☐ | ☐ | ☐ | ☐ |
| Beer | ☐ | ☐ | ☐ | ☐ | ☐ | ☐ |
| Wine | ☐ | ☐ | ☐ | ☐ | ☐ | ☐ |
| Wheat cereals/wheat products | ☐ | ☐ | ☐ | ☐ | ☐ | ☐ |
| Corn | ☐ | ☐ | ☐ | ☐ | ☐ | ☐ |
| Chocolate | ☐ | ☐ | ☐ | ☐ | ☐ | ☐ |
| Berries - strawberries/other_____ | ☐ | ☐ | ☐ | ☐ | ☐ | ☐ |
| Nut - Peanut/other_____ | ☐ | ☐ | ☐ | ☐ | ☐ | ☐ |
| Seafood-Shrimp/lobster/other_____ | ☐ | ☐ | ☐ | ☐ | ☐ | ☐ |
| Fish | ☐ | ☐ | ☐ | ☐ | ☐ | ☐ |
| Beef | ☐ | ☐ | ☐ | ☐ | ☐ | ☐ |
| Other food(s) _____ | ☐ | ☐ | ☐ | ☐ | ☐ | ☐ |

Allergy   Immunology Review

V.  Circle or complete the correct answers to describe your residence.

| | | | | |
|---|---|---|---|---|
| Type | House | Apartment | Condominium | Dormitory |
| Location | Seashore | City | Mountain | Desert |
| Age of Dwelling ___years | Years of occupancy _____ | | | |
| Bedroom Floor Coverings | Carpet | Wood | Cement | Linoleum |
| Bedroom Furniture | Overstuffed | Foam rubber | Antique | Other_____ |
| Pillows | Feather | Foam rubber | Dacron | |
| Indoor Animals | Cat | Dog | Bird | Other_____ |
| Outdoor Animals | Cat | Dog | Horse | Other_____ |

VI.  Circle characteristics or complete the blanks to describe yourself:

| | | |
|---|---|---|
| Financial problems | Major | Little |
| Nervous Tension | Considerable | Little |
| Work Adjustment | Easy | Difficult |
| School Adjustment | Easy | Difficult |
| Marital Adjustment | Easy | Difficult |

Year of last tetanus immunization _____

Year of last influenza immunization _____

Approximate date last took aspirin/or aspirin containing medication _____

Approximate date last took penicillin _____

Average hours of sleep per night _____

Packs of cigarettes smoked per day_____

Other tobacco per week _____

Bottles of beer per week_____

Alcoholic drinks per week _____

Hobbies _____

VII.  Treatment

| Treatment | Received | Helpful | Side effects |
|---|---|---|---|
| Antihistamines/decongestants | ☐ | ☐ | ☐ |
| Oral bronchodilators | ☐ | ☐ | ☐ |
| Inhaled medications | ☐ | ☐ | ☐ |
| Antibiotics | ☐ | ☐ | ☐ |
| Pollen, mold, dust injections | ☐ | ☐ | ☐ |
| Bacterial vaccines | ☐ | ☐ | ☐ |
| Food elimination | ☐ | ☐ | ☐ |

_____   _____

Patient's Signature                              Date

Physician Comment  (Circle on basis of history)

Conjunctivitis · Reagin   Irritant   Contact   Vernal

Rhinitis/Sinusitis · Reagin   Vasomotor  Mucoid  Purulent  Medicamentosa  Atrophic  Irritants

Asthma/Bronchitis · Reagin  p. viral  URI  Aspirin  Inhaler  Abuse  Irritant  Exercise  Mucoid
        Atmospheric change    Emotional    CHF    Esophageal Reflux    Carcinoid Occupational

Urticaria/Angioedema · Sporadic   Chronic · Food   Drug   Exercise   Heat   Cold
      Light   Emotional   Infection   Neoplasm   CT Disorder   Familial

Drug Reaction · Reagin    Other Immunologic    Non · Immunologic _____ (Drug)

Pruritus/Eczema · Reagin   Delayed contact sensitivity   Irritant   Neurodermatitis

Sting Insect · Reagin    Other

_____   _____

SCMG Physician's Signature                         Date

23

## REFERENCES

1. Mathison DA, Stevenson DD, Tan EM, et al: Clinical profiles of bronchial asthma. JAMA 224:1134–1139, 1973
2. Reed CA, Townley RG: Asthma, classification and pathogenesis, in Middleton E Jr, Reed CE, Ellis EF (Eds): Allergy, Principles and Practice. St. Louis, Mosby, 1978, pp 659–677
3. Solomon WR, Mathews KP: Aerobiology and inhalant allergens, in Middleton E Jr, Reed CE, Ellis EF (Eds): Allergy, Principles and Practice. St. Louis, Mosby, 1978, pp 929–964
4. Tovey ER, Chapman MD, Wells CW, et al: The distribution of dust mite allergen in the houses of patients with asthma. Am Rev Respir Dis 124:630–635, 1981
5. Lehrer SB, Wilson MR, Karr RM, Salvaggio JE: IgE antibody responses of smokers, non-smokers, and "smoke sensitive" persons to tobacco leaf and smoke antigens. Am Rev Respir Dis 121:168–170
6. Yodaken RE: The uncertain consequences of formaldehyde toxicity. JAMA 246:1677–1678, 1981
7. Zweiman B, Salvin RG, Reinberg RJ, et al: Effects of air pollution on asthma: A review. Allergy Clin Immunol 50:305–314, 1972
8. Wald ER, Milmoe GJ, Bowen A, et al: Acute maxillary sinusitis. N Engl J Med 304:749–754, 1981 (editorial on pp 779–780)
9. McFadden ER: Exercise-induced asthma. Am J Med 68:471–472, 1980
10. Reisman RE: Asthma induced by adrenergic aerosols. J Allergy 162–177, 1970
11. Mathison DA, Pleskow WW, Stevenson DD, et al: Aspirin and chemical sensitivities and challenges in asthmatic patients, in Spector SC (Ed): Provocative Challenge: Bronchial, Oral, Nasal and Exercise Procedures. Boca Raton, Fla, CRC Press, in press
12. Stevenson DD, Simon RA: Sensitivity to ingested metabisulfites in asthmatic subjects. J Allergy Clin Immunol 68:26–32, 1981
13. Berman SZ, Mathison DA, Stevenson DD, et al: Maxillary sinusitis and asthma. J Allergy Clin Immunol 53:311–317, 1974
14. Kjellen G, Tibbling L, Wranne B: Effect of conservative treatment of oesophageal dysfunction on bronchial asthma. Eur J Respir Dis 62:190–197, 1981
15. Rosenberg M, Patterson R, Mintzer R, et al: Clinical and immunologic criteria for the diagnosis of allergic bronchopulmonary aspergillosis. Ann Intern Med 86:405–414, 1977

# 3

ARTHUR DAWSON

# Examination of the Chest

## GENESIS OF THE RESPIRATORY SOUNDS

Considering how much time physicians spend listening to respiratory sounds, the standard texts of chest medicine contain remarkably little description of these sounds and even less discussion of their genesis and basic significance.

The normal breath sounds result from turbulent flow in the conducting airways. Some of the energy lost in accelerating eddy currents in the turbulent stream is converted to propagated vibrations that are conducted through the overlying lung parenchyma to the chest wall, where they can be heard with the stethoscope. Turbulence develops in gas flowing in a cylindrical tube such as a bronchus when the Reynolds number exceeds a critical value of about 1000:

$$\text{Reynolds number} = \frac{\text{linear velocity} \times \text{radius} \times \text{gas density}}{\text{gas viscosity}}$$

Therefore, we would expect to hear the breath sounds best over large-diameter airways where the linear velocity is high, which is indeed the case. Parenthetically, we would expect the sounds to diminish if we replaced air in the inspired gas with 80% helium in oxygen and to increase if we breathed a dense gas such as sulfur hexafluoride or if we entered a hyperbaric chamber. The first of these assumptions at least can readily be verified.

The breath sounds are relatively poorly heard at the lung bases because with each successive division of the conducting airways the total cross-sectional area increases and thus the linear velocity of the airflow in those airways diminishes. In addition, the alveoli are excellent sound insulators and the transmission to the chest wall of the sound of air movement in the conducting airways is markedly attenuated by the overlying parenchyma.

## Crackles

Rales, crackles, or crepitations are sounds produced when collapsed airways pop open during inspiratory lung expansion. They usually are heard at the bases because small airways tend to collapse in regions of high interstitial and hydrostatic pressure. They are accentuated if inspiration is preceded by a forced expiration.

## THE WHEEZE

The normal breath sounds and crackles create noise. A wheeze or rhonchus is a musical sound produced by a regularly oscillating element that generates organized vibrations of a harmonically related frequency. Wheezes are heard mainly during expiration and are characteristic of obstructive lung disease, especially bronchospasm.

The musical nature of the sound has suggested analogies to several musical instruments to account for the origin of wheezes. The oldest and least convincing explanation is that strands of mucus act like violin strings that are agitated by the flow of air. If this were so, it would be difficult to account for the occurrence of wheezes over the whole chest, their relatively constant frequency, and their failure to shift or disappear after coughing.

A somewhat more persuasive suggestion is that the sound is produced in a manner similar to a flute by air flowing past the orifice of an obstructed bronchus just as one can make a musical note by blowing over the mouth of a beer bottle. This theory is contradicted by the pitch of the sounds, which is much lower than can be generated by pipes of the few inches in length possible in an obstructed segment of bronchus. It is also denied by the observation that the pitch of a wheeze does not change when the inspired air is replaced with helium and oxygen while the frequency of sound produced by a wind instrument rises with a less dense gas.

Actually, it appears that wheezes are produced from a region of near collapse in a bronchus whose orifice rapidly oscillates between the closed and barely open position. Forgacs* suggests that the analogous musical instrument is a simple uncoupled reed similar to the detached mouthpiece of an aboe or the reed of a toy trumpet that can be shown to deliver a note whose frequency is unaffected by the density of the ambient gas.

### Why Do Some Asthmatics Have No Audible Wheeze?

Wheezing is a very consistent phenomenon in bronchospasm of moderate severity, but sometimes adventitious sounds are completely absent. For instance, when wheezing is absent in mild bronchospasm, it presumably means that the partial collapse of major airways has improved to the point where there are no remaining vibrating elements to generate musical sound. Spirometry may still demonstrate persistent bronchospasm. Also, when bronchial obstruction becomes more severe, the location of points of airways collapse tend to move "upstream" to smaller branches. These small airways probably cannot act effectively as the vibrating elements to generate musical sound. In very severe airways obstruction, bronchial mucus plugging may completely occlude and thereby silence the partially collapsed elements that previously generated sound.

Therefore, the diminution of wheezes may be a sign of improvement but can also be a manifestation of worsening of bronchial obstruction. In the latter case there is a simultaneous decrease in the intensity of the breath sounds. When wheezes disappear in a hospitalized patient without amelioration of respiratory distress, the physician should be

---

*As the author states: "Most textbooks of pulmonary diseases dismiss lung sounds in a few short paragraphs written in the language of the last century." This is a brief and readable introduction to twentieth century ideas about pulmonary sounds.

on guard. That may be the time to recheck the arterial blood gases. Valuable clues such as pulsus paradoxus may also be physical signs of severe airways obstruction.

Conversely, a patient admitted for the treatment of severe bronchospasm may show a marked augmentation of wheezes when the condition improves. Typically there will also be an increase in the intensity of the basal breath sounds, and the increased wheezing presumably reflects improved air entry and reversal of the phenomena of severe bronchial obstruction that tend to silence the musical sounds.

## PULSUS PARADOXUS

Pulsus paradoxus is not truly paradoxical. It is an augmentation of the normal tendency of the pulse pressure, systolic pressure, and stroke volume to diminish during inspiration and increase during expiration. Minor degrees of pulsus paradoxus can be detected by measuring with a sphygmomanometer the difference between inspiratory and expiratory systolic pressure, which should not exceed 8 mm Hg during quiet breathing. When marked, it can easily be appreciated by palpation of the arterial pulse.

Various explanations have been offered for pulsus paradoxus. It is known that during inspiration there is an increase in venous return to the right heart while lung expansion increases the capacity of the pulmonary vessels, thereby reducing venous return to the left heart. Much more important is the phenomenon of "interdependence" of the left and right ventricles. When right ventricular filling is augmented, not only its free wall, but also the interventricular septum is stretched. This stretching of the interventricular septum reduces the compliance of the left ventricle so that it can accept less venous return during diastole. The extreme case of interdependence of the ventricles occurs in cardiac tamponade when the sum of right and left ventricular end diastolic volumes is fixed. Therefore, any inspiratory augmentation of right ventricular filling is subtracted from the left ventricular stroke volume.

In obstructive lung disease the respiratory swings in intrathoracic pressure increase, and thus the respiratory variation in venous return to the right heart is greater than normal. Pulsus paradoxus results.

If pulsus paradoxus can be detected by palpation of the pulse, severe airways obstruction is indicated. It is in just this situation that wheezes may not be audible over the chest, and therefore careful examination of the pulse is of great importance in the bedside evaluation of patients with severe bronchospasm.

## EXAMINATION OF THE HEART

The heart sounds are produced by closure of the valves. The first sound is due to sudden tensing of the cusps and chordae of the mitral and tricuspid valves (mainly the mitral) as they reach the limit of their movement toward the atrial cavities. The second sound is produced by tensing of the cusps of the aortic and pulmonic valves.

In obstructive lung disease there can be striking respiratory variation of the intensity of the heart sounds. Presumably this variation results from the same mechanism as pulsus paradoxus, and the rapid augmentation of the heart sounds at the onset of inspiration suggests that most of the sound may arise in the right side of the heart rather than in the left as it normally does.

Another bedside sign of loading of the right heart in obstructive lung disease is a shift of the point of maximum impulse to the epigastrium. The epigastric pulsation may be especially prominent during inspiration. Its genesis is probably due to a combination of augmented right ventricular stroke volume and obscuring of the normal apical impulse by overinflation of the chest.

These physical signs are important because they may provide a clue to the presence of severe airways obstruction when the usual auscultatory findings in the chest are absent or misleading.

## THE CHEST RADIOGRAPH

It certainly is advisable to obtain a chest film on a patient newly presenting with asthma or complaining of markedly worsening symptoms, but the study is usually uninformative, and there seems to be little excuse for the common practice of getting a chest film and neglecting the far more useful spirogram. The chest film may turn up unexpected pneumonia or an obstructing bronchial tumor in a wheezing patient or even a spontaneous pneumothorax, but generally the study is helpful only to rule out such problems. On careful inspection the film may show downward displacement of the diaphragms, narrowing of the peripheral vessels and reduction of the heart size, all manifestations of increased lung volume and a high alveolar pressure during expiration, but these signs are too nonspecific and subjective to be of much diagnostic value.

## REFERENCE

1.   Forgacs P: The functional basis of pulmonary sounds. Chest 73:399–405, 1978

# 4

DAVID A. MATHISON

# Examination of Upper Respiratory Tract and Evaluation of Respiratory Secretions

## PHYSICAL EXAMINATION

Optimal physical examination of the nose, paranasal sinuses, pharynx, ear canals, and tympanic membranes requires a lamp, head mirror, nasal speculum, sinus transilluminator, and pneumatic otoscope. The nose should be examined after shrinkage of the nasal membranes with a sympathomimetic agent and application of a topical anesthetic. Such an examination is best performed by an otorhinolaryngologist. Practical examination in the office or at the bedside can be accomplished with an otoscope with nasal-size tip, sinus transilluminator, and tongue blade.

The nasal mucous membranes ordinarily are paler than the conjunctival and oral membranes. When vasomotor rhinitis or an immediate hypersensitivity reaction causes edema of the nasal membranes, there is a pale slate-blue discoloration and engorgement, especially over the turbinates. Overuse of sympathomimetic nasal drops or sprays (rhinitis medicamentosus) and acute viral illness produce erythematous edema. Yellow mucopurulent secretions are found in the presence of bacterial infection and in eosinophilic exudates of immediate hypersensitivity, aspirin sensitivity, and other non-IgE eosinophilic states. Microscopic examination of the secretion helps to distinguish these conditions. Dry, crusted, atrophic membranes are found in the sicca-atrophy syndromes.

The frontal and maxillary sinuses transilluminate poorly or not at all if there is mucoperiosteal thickening, polypoid change, fluid, or mucocele in the sinus. Transillumination may also be reduced if the bony walls of the sinuses are unusually thick and dense or if an upper denture has not been removed by the patient.

## SINUS ROENTGENOGRAMS

Four view sinus roentgenograms (Fig. 4-1) should be done in asthmatic patients if there are upper respiratory symptoms or if the sinuses do not transilluminate, but they must be interpreted with caution. Mucoperiosteal thickening of more than a few millimeters is found in approximately 20% of normal individuals, whereas 50% of asthmatic patients[1] have this or some other abnormality. The finding of an air fluid level (Fig. 4-2) or complete opacification (Fig. 4-3) in one or more of the paranasal sinuses

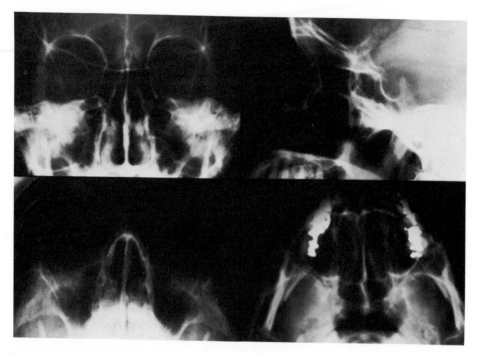

**Fig. 4-1.** Posterior-anterior (top left), lateral (top right), Water's (lower left), and basal (lower right) roentgenograms of normal sinuses.

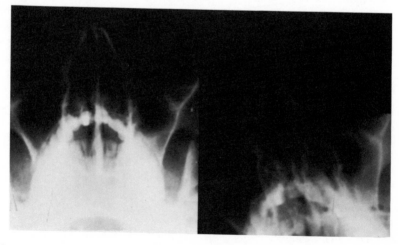

**Fig. 4-2.** Roentgenograms of acute left maxillary sinusitis (Water's, left), including confirmation of fluid shift in lateral decubitus view (right).

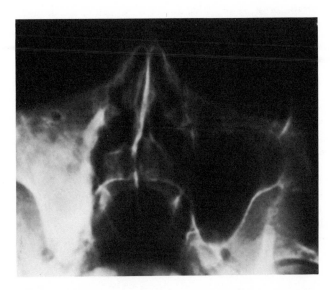

**Fig. 4-3.** Opacified right maxillary sinus (Water's view); differential diagnosis includes bacterial sinusitis, polypoid filling, and sinus tumor.

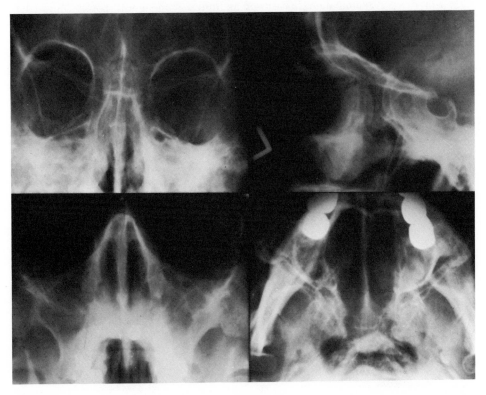

**Fig. 4-4.** Parasinusitis with clouding of frontal-ethmoid (top left), splenoid (top right), and maxillary (bottom left and right) sinuses.

strongly suggests the presence of active microbial sinusitis, which may contribute to the asthma. Mucoperiosteal thickening, polypoid changes, or opacification in the maxillary, ethmoid, and frontal sinuses (Fig. 4-4) should raise a suspicion of aspirin sensitivity.

## NASAL SECRETIONS

Microscopic examination of the cells in a nasal smear provides clues as to the nature and origin of nasal inflammation. The technique for collection and staining of the specimen is as follows:

1.  Swab—swirl a cotton-tipped wire nasal applicator (Caligswab®) through nose from the anterior nares, along the inferior turbinate to the nasopharynx and back.
2.  Roll the applicator over a microscope slide and immediately fix in 95% ethanol for several minutes.
3.  Cover the slide with Wright Giemsa stain—Hansel modification (Hansel Stain-Lide Labs, Inc., St. Louis) for 30–60 seconds.
4.  Add 2–3 drops of distilled water, mix with stain, and allow to stand for 30–60 seconds.
5.  Rinse with distilled water and allow to dry in air or under a fan.

Microscopic examination consists of an initial scan at low power followed by high-power viewing to identify cell types. Finally the slide is examined under oil immersion to detect microbes. Cells that can be identified include (1) normal cylindric or stellate respiratory epithelial cells that are often clumped, (2) eosinophils with their bilobed nuclei and large red cytoplasmic granules, (3) neutrophils with their multilobed

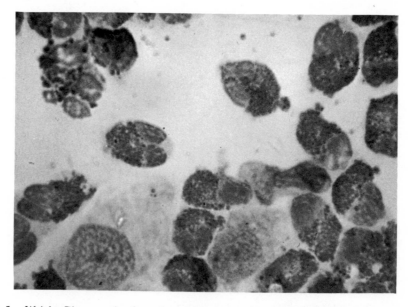

**Fig. 4-5.** Wright-Giemsa stain of nasal secretions (original × 100 magnification) shows predominance of eosinophils, several epithelial cells (lower), and mast cell (top left).

nuclei and pale cytoplasmic granules, (4) basophils and mast cells that are usually larger than eosinophils and have coarse metachromatic reddish-purple football-shaped granules (histamine-heparin) that obscure the nucleus, (5) goblet cells that are foamy-appearing, and (6) mucus-secreting cells most often seen in association with eosinophils or mast cells.

When basophils or mast cells and eosinophils (Fig. 4-5) are found in the nasal secretions, the mediators of immediate hypersensitivity—including histamine and eosinophil chemotactic factor of anaphylaxis—are likely to account for the inflammation.

When one finds ciliocytophoric changes of the epithelial cells (margination of nuclear chromatin, nuclear pyknosis, or broken off ciliated tufts, acute viral infection is implicated as the source of inflammation. The presence of neutrophils in association with bacteria suggests active bacterial infection. Occasionally the hyphae of Aspergillus or the yeast forms of *Candida albicans* can be recognized.

Pathogenic bacteria cultured from nasal-nasopharyngeal swabs of patients with purulent (i.e., neutrophils on smear) rhinitis-sinusitis or pharyngitis ordinarily are considered to have pathophysiologic significance. Samples obtained from puncture irrigation of the maxillary antra or at the time of sinus surgery should be Gram-stained and cultured for anaerobic and aerobic bacteria, fungi, and acid-fast organisms. *Haemophilus influenzae, Streptococcus pneumoniae,* and anaerobic bacteria are the microorganisms most frequently recovered in acute illness.[2]

## SPUTUM AND TRACHEOBRONCHIAL SECRETIONS

Gross examination of the volume and contents of sputum collected over a 24-hour period provides clues as to the nature and intensity of tracheobronchial inflammation. In patients with acute or persistent asthmatic relapse, adequate clearing of secretions may be prevented by bronchospasm and edema, and usually there is only scanty colorless or mucoid sputum. Yellow-colored sputum is found in eosinophilic or neutrophilic secretions, but color alone does not discriminate bacterial from other varieties of inflammation. Patients who have had weeks or months of asthmatic relapse gradually clear a couple of ounces daily of mucoid secretions, including mustard seed-sized brown bronchial casts as they respond to adequate bronchodilator, corticosteroid, and pulmonary toilet measures. In the modern era of corticosteroid treatment of asthma, asthmatic patients only occasionally produce casts of the larger airways recognized as "kite stings" several centimeters long or Curschmann's spirals. Malodorous, purulent layering sputum reflects bacterial bronchitis or bronchiectasis sometimes associated with asthma.

Strands or flecks of dense material from fresh sputum[3] or tracheobronchial aspirate are the best materials for cultures and examination of sputum cells. Gram stains allow preliminary identification of bacteria and polymorphonuclear inflammatory cells and also can be used to determine whether the specimen came from the upper respiratory tract. The Gram stain does not readily distinguish neutrophils from eosinophils. The Wright-Giemsa stain–Hansel modification (as used for nasal secretions) or buffered crystal violet stain allow identification of eosinophils and their debris, the elongated double pyramidal crystals described by Charcot-Leyden. The presence of eosinophils or Charcot-Leyden crystals in tracheal-bronchial secretions is virtually diagnostic of asthma. Examination and culture of a smear for fungi is important for the diagnosis of bronchopulmonary Aspergillosis. Further details of sputum analysis in general are described by Washington.[3] Further information on the examination of sputum cells can be found in an article by Chodosh.[4]

## REFERENCES

1. Berman SZ, Mathison DA, Stevenson DD, et al: Maxillary sinusitis and bronchial asthma: Correlations of roentgenograms, cultures, and thermograms. J Allergy Clin Immunol 53:311–317, 1974
2. Wold ER, Milmoe GJ, Bowen A, et al: Acute maxillary sinusitis. New Engl J Med 304:749–754, 1981 (editorial, pp 779–780)
3. Washington JA: Maximizing diagnostic yield from sputum examination. J Respir Dis 2:81–92, 1981
4. Chodosh S: Sputum cytology in chronic bronchial disease. Adv Allergy Pulm Dis 4:8, 1977

# 5

DAVID A. MATHISON

# Cutaneous and Other Tests for Immediate Hypersensitivity

Immunologic responses to exogenous or autologous substances sometimes initiate chemical mediator and effector cell responses that are more intense than necessary to protect the host from the antigen and that lead to injury of the host. Diseases that can be attributed to immunopathologic injury are termed "allergic," "immunologic," "hyperimmune," or, when autologous antigens initiate the immune response, "autoimmune." Two decades ago Coombs and Gell[1] conveniently classified these disorders by the nature of the immunologic component to include anaphylactic or immediate hypersensitivity reactions (Type I), tissue or cell lytic reactions (Type II), immune complex reactions (Type III), and reactions mediated by specific sensitized lymphocytes (Type IV) (Table 5-1). Although knowledge of the nature of antigens, antibodies, and the dynamics of cellular and molecular interactions that account for the immunologic-inflammatory response has greatly expanded in the intervening years, the Gell-Coombs classification remains a useful reference point.

Asthma can be attributed to an immediate hypersensitivity (IgE-mediated) reaction to aeroallergens when the history (see Chapter 2) links exacerbations to exposures to pollens, dust mite, spores, or animals, and cutaneous or serum tests confirm the presence of IgE antibodies to the putative aeroallergens. It is reasonable to presume the role of IgE antibodies in "allergic" or "extrinsic" asthma when the history is typical of reactivity to pollen or animal protein and when the asthma is mild and readily controlled by simple medication or avoidance measures. When the asthma problem is more complicated and the history more equivocal for an IgE reaction, as with sensitivity to dust mite and spores, or when immunotherapy is contemplated, tests for specific IgE antibodies are indicated. Since less than 1% of the specific and total IgE antibodies are free in the serum, with the rest affixed to cutaneous and other mast cells, cutaneous tests ordinarily provide more useful information than do tests of serum.

Direct cutaneous tests for specific IgE antibodies are performed with aqueous extracts of dried whole crude materials applied either in concentrated form to pinprick disruptions of the skin (prick—qualitative) or in a series increasing concentrations injected into the dermis (intradermal—semiquantitative). Details of these methods are described by Vanselow.[2] Fifteen-minute wheal reactions are interpreted and compared to a positive control test with histamine and a negative control test with the saline-phenol preservative.

Figure 5-1 shows exemplary test results from an asthmatic patient with a history of

**Table 5-1**

**Summary of Coombs and Gel Classification of Immunopathologic Reactions**

| Type of Reaction | Antibody Involved | Complement Involved | Mediators of Injury | Clinical Examples | Test |
|---|---|---|---|---|---|
| I. Anaphylactic | IgE | None | Histamine SRS-A Eosinophils | Hay fever Asthma | Cutaneous 15 minute Wheal and Flare RAST |
| II. Membranolytic | IgG or IgM | C1–9 | Complement lysis | Transfusion reaction Good pasture's syndrome | Serologic for antibody |
| III. Immune complex | IgG or IgM | C3, C5 Chemotactic factors | Polymorphonuclear leukocytes | Serum sickness Systemic lupus Erythematosus | Serologic for antibody–immune complex |
| IV. Delayed (cell mediated) | None | None | Lymphocytes Lymphokines Macrophages | Contact dermatitis Allograft or tumor rejection | Delayed (48–72 h) cutaneous reaction |

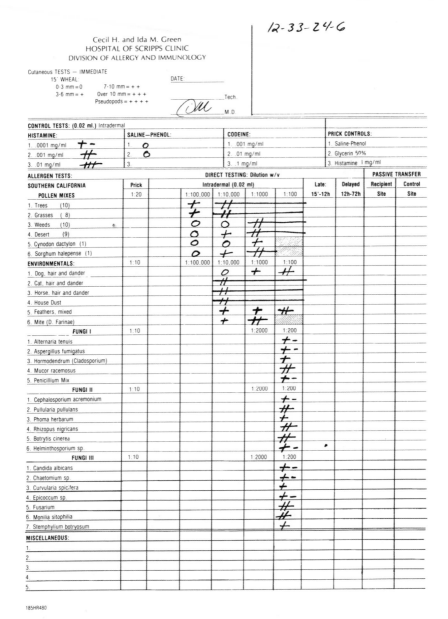

**Fig. 5-1.** Test results from patient with perennial asthma: seasonal exacerbation in spring and sporadic exacerbations following exposure to cats and dust mite.

perennial disease with a notable seasonal exacerbation in the spring and sporadic exacerbations after exposure to cats and to house dust. The tests in this case confirmed the presence of high titers of IgE antibodies to tree and grass pollens (spring) and to cat and in moderate titers to dust mite. The tests also suggest modest titers of IgE to dog, feathers, and several mold spore extracts, but in the absence of any history suggesting a reaction on natural exposures, these IgE antibodies were not judged to have clinical relevance.

If the history suggests the presence of immediate hypersensitivity but tests for IgE antibody are negative, immediate hypersensitivity is virtually excluded as a contributing factor to the asthma.

As most grass pollens and many weed pollens cross-react in their allergenicity, mixtures of grass and weed pollens may be used for cutaneous tests, reducing the number of injections that need to be done. Cross-allergenicity is less common among tree pollens, but in most areas no more than a half-dozen tree species account for the great majority of relevant allergens. Fungus species have little cross-reactivity and vary greatly in their ability to act as allergens. Those species listed as "Fungi I" in Figure 1 most frequently account for disease in southern California; species listed in "Fungi II" are less frequently significant, and "Fungi III" are still less frequently important.

Direct cutaneous tests for IgE antibodies are the most sensitive, least expensive, and most readily performed (at least by the allergist) and are available for the greatest numbers of allergens. In vitro tests include radioallergosorbent (RAST) tests of serum,[3] tests performed following the passive transfer of serum to a nonsensitive human's skin (Prausnitz-Kustner or PK reaction), and tests of leukocyte histamine release. RAST tests are required for individuals with generalized dermatitis or dermographism when direct testing cannot be done and are performed by the technique shown in Figure 5-2. The

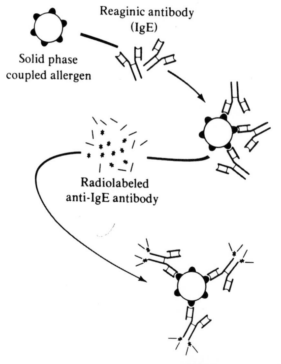

**Fig. 5-2.**   Radioallergosorbent test (RAST): allergen is covalently bound to solid phase. Patient serum sample containing specific IgE antibody is incubated with solid phase. Radiolabeled anti-IgE antibody is added and attaches to IgE antibody–allergen–solid-phase proportionate to amount of IgE antibody. Solid-phase reactants are separated from liquid-phase unbound radiolabeled anti-IgE and counted.

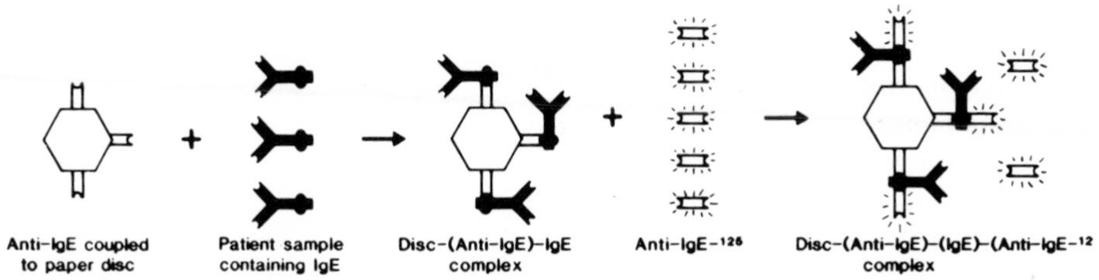

Anti–IgE coupled to paper disc · Patient sample containing IgE · Disc–(Anti–IgE)–IgE complex · Anti–IgE-¹²⁵ · Disc–(Anti–IgE)–(IgE)–(Anti–IgE-¹²) complex

**Fig. 5-3.** PRIST (Pharmacia Diagnostics) test: anti-IgE is convalently coupled to paper disk. Patient serum containing IgE is incubated with the coated disks and produces disk–anti-IgE–IgE complex. After washing, radioactivity labeled, immunosorbent purified anti-IgE antibodies are added. Solid-phase reactants are separated from liquid-phase unbound radiolabeled anti-IgE and counted.

results are scored in a semiquantitive fashion as follows:

Score 0 = negative, no IgE antibodies
Score 1 = borderline, very low levels of IgE antibodies
Score 2 = low levels of IgE antibodies
Score 3 = moderate levels of IgE antibodies
Score 4 = very high levels of IgE antibodies

Approximately 20% of a population without respiratory disease has specific IgE

**Table 5-2**
**Expected Phadebas IgE PRIST Levels***
**U.S. Population Study†**

| Age | Subjects (N=) | Geometric Mean IgE U/ml | Geometric Mean ±1 SD IgE U/ml |
|---|---|---|---|
| Newborn | 37 | 0.53 | 0.27–1.04 |
| 1–11 mo | 51 | 2.45 | 0.51–11.75 |
| 1 yr | 22 | 2.74 | 0.50–15.08 |
| 2 yr | 26 | 6.18 | 1.33–28.66 |
| 3 yr | 33 | 11.83 | 4.05–34.54 |
| 4 yr | 27 | 7.44 | 1.69–32.71 |
| 5 yr | 30 | 21.00 | 7.90–55.84 |
| 6 yr | 31 | 15.79 | 2.62–95.10 |
| 7 yr | 30 | 13.97 | 2.22–87.82 |
| 8 yr | 32 | 18.84 | 4.97–71.38 |
| 9 yr | 35 | 16.52 | 3.12–87.53 |
| 10 yr | 40 | 28.48 | 7.41–109.51 |
| 11–14 yr | 98 | 26.89 | 6.53–110.76 |
| 15–19 yr | 50 | 24.23 | 6.08–96.48 |
| 20–30 yr | 52 | 14.37 | 3.52–58.67 |
| 31–50 yr | 52 | 19.38 | 4.74–79.27 |
| 51–80 yr | 34 | 11.79 | 2.88–48.24 |

*Correlates with Phadezym IgE PRIST.
†Data on file Pharmacia Diagnostics.

antibodies as determined by positive cutaneous or RAST tests to at least one common aeroallergen, and approximately 5–10% of a general population will react to any one of the common aeroallergens. The mere presence of a positive test, therefore, even in high titer, does not imply clinical relevance in a given patient. The test must be interpreted in relation to the history of exacerbations and environmental exposure.

Some practicioners attempt to use measurements of the total serum IgE to estimate the likelihood that IgE-mediated reactions contribute to asthma. Total serum IgE is best measured by a double anti-IgE antibody technique such as the paper radioimmunosorbent test (PRIST [Pharmacia Diagnostics, Piscataway, NJ]) illustrated in Fig. 5-3. Table 5-2 lists the geometric mean levels for PRIST IgE in normal persons at various ages. Asthmatic populations have statistical means that fall above the normal means, but interpretation of the meaning of serum IgE level for the individual asthmatic patient is more difficult. A normal, even a low normal, level does not exclude the presence of specific IgE that may be relevant, and a high level gives no information about specific antibodies or whether they are clinically significant. A very high ($>2000$ IU/ml) level should increase suspicion for bronchopulmonary aspergillosis (see Chapter 2).

In summary, when the asthma is complicated and the history inconclusive or when immunotherapy is planned, the patient should be tested by direct prick (qualitative) or intradermal (semiquantitative) cutaneous methods selective for a wheal–flare response indicative of specific IgE antibodies directed against aeroallergens. When tests confirm that there are IgE antibodies to aeroallergens in the home environment that could be relevant to the asthma, avoidance measures should be used when possible. Immunotherapy (desensitization) is sometimes indicated for those aeroallergens that contribute to the asthma and that cannot be avoided (see Chapter 16).

## REFERENCES

1.   Coombs RRA, Gell PGH: The classification of allergic reactions underlying diseases, in Gell PGH, Coombs RRA (Eds): Clinical Aspects of Immunology, Philadelphia, Davis, 1962, pp. 313–377
2.   Vanselow NA: Skin testing and other diagnostic procedures, in Sheldon JM, Lovell RG, Mathews KP (Eds): A Manual of Clinical Allergy, Philadelphia, Saunders, 1967, pp 55–66
3.   Evans R: Advances in diagnosis of allergy: RAST. Symposia Specialists, Miami, 1975 (available from Pharmacia Diagnostics)

# 6

ARTHUR DAWSON

# Spirometry

The characteristic feature of bronchospasm is variable obstruction to respiratory airflow. It is not difficult for a physician to diagnose asthma when the patient complains of attacks of cough and wheeze and when auscultation of the chest shows high-pitched rhonchi. Some asthmatics provide a confusing or misleading history, however, and it is possible for a patient with quite severe bronchospasm to show no adventitious sounds on chest auscultation. Also, it is often difficult to judge from the bedside evaluation whether the patient has responded to treatment or whether there is any residual bronchial obstruction after acute symptoms have subsided.

For these reasons, it is essential for accurate diagnosis and successful treatment of bronchospasm to have some objective means of assessing the severity of bronchial obstruction. This is provided by spirometry.

Unfortunately, spirometry is a much underused diagnostic test. Many physicians are confused by the arcane terminology on the reports from pulmonary physiology laboratories and believe that the results obtained by this method can be interpreted only by a hospital laboratory or a specialist. Also, many laboratories charge far more than is appropriate to perform spirometry, so this method becomes too expensive to be used repeatedly as a guide to the patient's progress.

In fact, "limited" spirometry is a very simple technique that should be available in the office of any physician managing asthmatic patients—that is, all internists and family practitioners. The equipment is comparable in price with an electrocardiograph, and any office assistant who can operate an ECG machine should be able to learn to perform spirometry.

We shall not attempt to provide details on how to perform the test, calculate the results, and interpret the findings here. We will present a brief summary of spirometry to prepare the reader for interpretation of the data and flow–volume curves that are encountered in several other chapters.

## EQUIPMENT

The simplest and most reliable spirometer is the conventional volumetric device. The patient blows into a tube connected to a bell or bellows that is mechanically coupled with a pen. The pen records the volume change on a moving kymograph. The water spirometer is the device sanctioned by tradition, but several reliable "dry" or bellows spirometers have been shown to be just as accurate.

With such a spirometer the forced vital capacity (FVC) and 1-second forced expiratory volume ($FEV_1$) can be read off rapidly and reported without further calculation. If preferred, a programmable hand-held calculator with stable memory (i.e., programs are remembered when the power is turned off) can be purchased for about $100 and used to correct the directly measured volumes for room temperature and to calculate the predicted values for sex, age, and height. A suitable spirometer and calculator probably will cost around $1500.

The calculations can be performed much more rapidly, and an attractive report can be generated with one of the increasing number of microcomputer-based spirometry systems now appearing on the market. Those now available still cost in the $5000–$8000 range, probably more than any individual physician would be prepared to spend. However, the price of such devices is diminishing rapidly and it is only a matter of time before some enterprising company produces a digital spirometer suitable for the private medical office.

Most of the available electronic spirometers measure flow rather than volume; volume is calculated by integrating the flow signal. The accuracy of the device depends very much on the performance and calibration of the flow transducer. Unfortunately, it is only recently that adequate performance criteria for spirometric instruments have been established, and a number of spirometers sold a few years ago failed miserably in meeting the standards. Although these devices are no longer sold, some of them are still in use in physician's offices and even in hospital laboratories.

The newer microprocessor-based devices are more reliable, not only because manufacturing standards have improved, but also because microprocessors are much less subject to the problems of zero drift and electrical instability that plagued the older analog systems. Nevertheless, one cannot simply plug an electronic spirometer into the wall and expect it to perform reliably month after month without even a calibration check. The newer instruments can be easily calibrated, usually by injecting into them a known volume of air from a large syringe.

## CALCULATIONS

For those not initiated into the mysteries of lung physiology, spirometry has been needlessly complicated by the variety of spirometric indices that can be calculated from the curve relating forced expiratory volume to time. The terms used to describe certain indices have changed over the years, and in the last decade there has been a bewildering explosion of new information about "large" airways and "small" airways disease. For our purposes we need to calculate only two numbers:

1. The forced vital capacity or FVC is the total volume of air that can be expired during a forced expiration from full lung inflation.
2. The 1-second forced expiratory volume or $FEV_1$ is the volume of air expired during the first second of the forced expiratory maneuver. The $FEV_1$ can be expressed as a percentage of the FVC (abbreviated $FEV_1\%$), and it should be greater than 75% (or 70% in patients over age 40).

This information is sufficient for office follow-up of patients with brochospasm but for the purpose of illustration, we present the data in graphic form. Figure 6-1 shows the volume–time format.

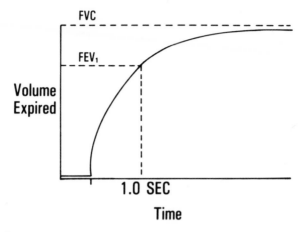

**Fig. 6-1.** A normal spirogram presented in the volume–time format.

The same information can be presented by plotting expiratory flow versus the volume expired. This is the flow–volume curve (Fig. 6-2), and although it must be stressed that it contains no different information, it does make it easier to identify mild bronchial obstruction.

Since the flow–volume curve has no time scale, neither the $FEV_1$ nor the total duration of expiration can be measured directly from it, but the $FEV_1$ can be represented by a "tic" on the curve.

## INTERPRETATION

Figure 6-3 demonstrates a normal flow–volume curve contrasted with a typical curve demonstrating moderate bronchial obstruction. Figure 6-4 gives, for purposes of comparison, the curve of a patient with restrictive disease without obstruction. Figure 6-5

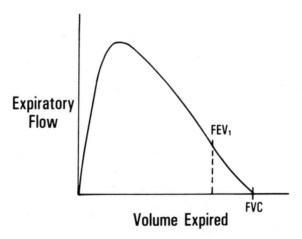

**Fig. 6-2.** A normal spirogram in the flow–volume format.

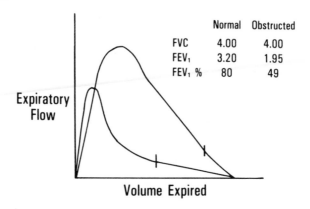

|  | Normal | Obstructed |
|---|---|---|
| FVC | 4.00 | 4.00 |
| $FEV_1$ | 3.20 | 1.95 |
| $FEV_1$ % | 80 | 49 |

**Fig. 6-3.** A normal flow–volume curve compared with one showing moderate airways obstruction.

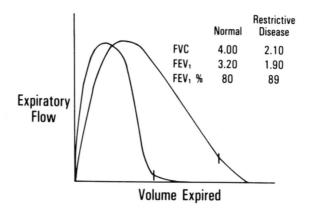

|  | Normal | Restrictive Disease |
|---|---|---|
| FVC | 4.00 | 2.10 |
| $FEV_1$ | 3.20 | 1.90 |
| $FEV_1$ % | 80 | 89 |

**Fig. 6-4.** A normal flow–volume curve compared with one showing moderate restrictive disease.

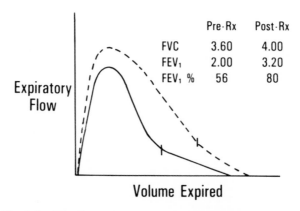

|  | Pre-Rx | Post-Rx |
|---|---|---|
| FVC | 3.60 | 4.00 |
| $FEV_1$ | 2.00 | 3.20 |
| $FEV_1$ % | 56 | 80 |

**Fig. 6-5.** The flow–volume curve of an asthmatic patient before (solid line) and after (dashed line) the administration of a bronchodilator aerosol.

**Table 6-1**
**Interpretation of Spirogram Results**

| Observed Value as Percent of Predicted, % | Interpretation |
|---|---|
| >80 | Probably normal |
| 65–80 | Mildly reduced |
| 50–64 | Moderately reduced |
| <50 | Severely reduced |

demonstrates the typical appearance of an asthmatic patient tested before and after treatment with a bronchodilator drug.

As a rough rule of thumb, the spirogram can be considered normal if the FVC and $FEV_1$ are greater than 80% of the predicted value and if the $FEV_1$% is 75% or more (70% in patients above age 40). Low values can be interpreted according to the scale shown in Table 6-1. The $FEV_1$ taken alone gives a rough guide to the severity of bronchial obstruction, and it may help to remember the figures presented in Table 6-2. The flow–volume curve of a patient with far-advanced emphysema would resemble the curve shown in Figure 6-6.

## CAN THE SPIROGRAM BE NORMAL IN THE PRESENCE OF ASTHMA?

When there is considerable bronchial mucus plugging, the spirogram may still appear normal or nearly so. It should be kept in mind that the predicted normal range of values is very large, and a patient who should have a supernormal test may fall within normal limits even during a symptomatic period. The reason for a normal-appearing curve is that completely obstructed airways cause a rise in the lung residual volume but no significant decrease in flow since no flow occurs through completely plugged airways. Sometimes the response to the bronchodilator will reveal the state of affairs (Fig. 6-7), but even this response may not be reliable because if the bronchial obstruction results from mucosal edema and mucus plugging rather than muscle spasm, there may be little change after the administration of a short-acting bronchodilator. In such cases it is useful for physicians to have spirometry in their offices and to record a baseline spirogram, just as they would record an electrocardiogram at the time when they accumulate the initial "data

**Table 6-2**
**$FEV_1$ as Index of Bronchial Obstruction**

| $FEV_1$ Liters | Clinical Correlation |
|---|---|
| 3.0–4.5 | Average normal adult values |
| 1.5–2.5 | Mild to moderate obstruction |
| <1.0 | Qualify for handicapped parking bumper sticker in California |
| <0.75 | Total disability |
| 0.4–0.6 | Values in patients with severe emphysema |

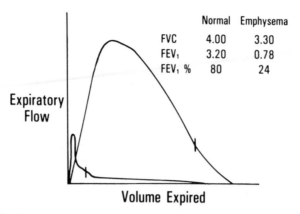

**Fig. 6-6.**  A normal flow-volume curve compared with that of a patient with severe pulmonary emphysema.

base." During even a mild attack of asthma, the spirometric measurements may fall within the broad limits of normal, but they will always be decreased from those recorded when the patient's bronchospasm is cleared.

## SPIROMETRY AS A GUIDE TO THERAPY

Spirometry is one of the most valuable ways to assess the patient's response to treatment. It should be kept in mind that for many patients with chronic bronchospasm, the occurrence of symptoms is only "the tip of the iceberg," and they may be perfectly comfortable even when they have a good deal of obstruction. The sequence shown in Figure 6-8 illustrates this point. This young man had a long history of mild asthma. He was seen 3 months after what appeared to be a minor viral respiratory infection complaining of persistent wheezing severe enough to prevent sleep. He had also lost 15 pounds. Examination showed wheezes over the whole chest. His spirogram is shown in Figure 6-8A before and after inhalation of isoetharine solution (Bronkosol [Breon

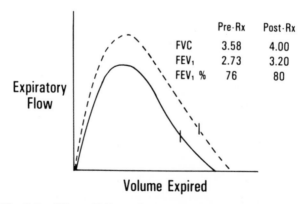

**Fig. 6-7.**  "Normal" flow-volume curves in an asthmatic patient before (solid line) and after (dashed line) the administration of a bronchodilator aerosol.

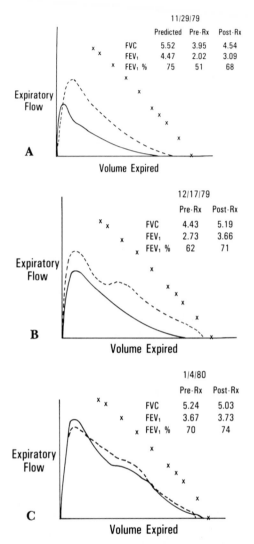

**6-8.** (A) Flow-volume curves of a patient with bronchial asthma in relapse prior to corticosteroid therapy, before (solid line), and after (dashed line) administration of a broncho-dilator aerosol. The predicated values are represented by the crosses. (B) The same patient after two weeks on prednisone. He is subjectively free of bronchospasm but the spirometry demonstrates substantial reversible bronchial obstruction. He will probably relapse if the prednisone is tapered at this point. (C) The same patient after a month of prednisone therapy. He is now free of reversible obstruction and successful withdrawl from prednisone is more likely.

Laboratories Inc., New York, NY]). He was begun on prednisone 30 mg/day and returned in 2 weeks. His wheeze and cough had disappeared, and he had regained 6 pounds. Auscultation of the chest was normal. His spirometry, shown in Figure 6-8B, reveals much improvement, but there is still considerable residual bronchospasm. In my experience, if tapering of the prednisone is begun at this point, symptoms are likely to recur. After another 2 weeks on the full dose of prednisone he returned still feeling well. Physical examination remained normal. At this time the spirometry showed no residual bronchospasm, and the prednisone was successfully withdrawn over the succeeding two weeks. He remained free of symptoms on theophylline by mouth and inhaled beclomethasone without further systemic corticosteroid therapy.

In summary, spirometry is necessary for the identification of bronchospasm and to assess the patient's response to treatment. Physicians regularly treating asthmatics (i.e., most internists and family practitioners) should have a spirometer in their offices.

## SUGGESTED READINGS

American Thoracic Society: Standardization of spirometry. Am Rev Respir Dis 119:831–838, 1979.
Kanner RE, Morris AH: Clinical Pulmonary Function Testing, Spirometry Intermountain Thoracic Society, Salt Lake City, 1975, Chapter 1
  *Detailed instructions on how to perform spirometry with the Collins Water Sealed Spirometer. Most of the instructions are applicable to other instruments.*
Morris JF: Spirometry in the evaluation of pulmonary function. West J Med 125:110–118, 1976
  *A brief and informative review including some references for predicted values.*

# 7

DAVID A. MATHISON

# Bronchial Provocations and Challenge Testing

To establish diagnoses of asthma, one must consider more than patients' descriptions of their symptoms. A method to assess the severity and degree of reversibility of the airway obstruction must be required. Patients commonly complain of labored breathing accompanied by wheezing and a sense of chest constriction and, often, of attacks of coughing and gasping due to interference with airflow in and out of the lungs. Physiologically, the hallmark of asthma is increased responsiveness of the trachea and bronchi to various stimuli, that is, bronchial hyperactivity. The result is widespread narrowing of the airways that is reversible—either spontaneously, or following bronchodilator therapy.

Changes in airway narrowing are most frequently documented, and the diagnosis confirmed, by spirometric measurements showing an improvement in forced expiratory volume or flow following the inhalation of a bronchodilator (see Chapter 6). Although it is not ordinarily regarded in such terms, this kind of inhalation "challenge" is a time-honored method of making the diagnosis of asthma.

Due to the paroxysmal nature of asthma, it may not be possible to demonstrate reversible airway obstruction when the patient is in remission or when symptoms are minimal or atypical. Some asthmatics, for example, complain of attacks of cough rather than wheezing and dyspnea. In such instances, asthmatic bronchospasm may be identified by a provocative challenge with inhaled methacholine or histamine or with strenuous exercise.

## METHACHOLINE CHALLENGE

When simple spirometry fails to establish the presence of reversible obstruction and the patient's baseline $FEV_1$ (forced expiratory volume in one second) is 80% or more of the predicted or highest previously observed value, methacholine challenge may be tried. Methacholine produces reflex and direct bronchoconstrictive responses in the asthmatic patient. If the patient has already received an inhaled bronchodilator, the challenge should be postponed for 2 hours to allow its effects to subside.

Aerosols of methacholine are delivered through a glass nebulizer connected to a source of compressed air, which permits the patient to activate the delivery of a precise volume of aerosol. Methacholine chloride is diluted in buffered saline (pH 7.0) containing

0.4% phenol. Concentrations of 5 and 25 mg/ml are used for qualitative determinations; for quantitative dose-response challenges, concentrations of 0.075, 0.15, 0.31, 0.62, 1.25, 2.5, 5.0, 10.0, and 25.0 mg/ml are used.

The qualitative test is performed by giving a single maximum inhalation of the 5-mg/ml methacholine, following baseline duplicate spirometry. If there is a less than 20% fall in the $FEV_1$, the process is repeated with another inhalation at 25 mg/ml; if there is still a fall of less than 20%, four additional inhalations of 25 mg/ml each are administered. If a fall greater than 20% occurs, the test is considered positive and the airway obstruction is reversed with aerosolized 0.5% isoproterenol solution 0.5 ml in 2.5 ml of water.

Figure 7-1 shows the response of a mildly asthmatic patient to such a challenge. Figure 7-2 shows the result of qualitative methacholine challenge in 121 adults with a history of asthma (defined by shortness of breath accompanied by wheezing and a sensation of chest constriction) and in 20 adults with no respiratory disease.

All groups of patients with asthma have a similar distribution of reactivity to methacholine. The subgroups include patients who have experienced exacerbations attributable to aeroallergens, aspirin sensitivity, exercise, and exposure to irritants.

Approximately 40% of patients with chronic bronchitis (defined by recurrent productive cough or best $FEV_1$ of less than 60% of predicted value) will also react to methacholine. For such patients, a diagnosis of asthmatic bronchitis is appropriate and treatment with a bronchodilator should be considered.

The qualitative methacholine challenge can be performed in most patients over age 6. However, it may provoke a severe asthmatic response and should not be used in patients with active asthma or patients who are known to have moderate to severe obstructive or restrictive bronchopulmonary disease. Patients with severe obstructive airway disease whose $FEV_1$ is less than 1.5 liters may develop severe respiratory distress following even a small change in the $FEV_1$. These patients, as well as those whose $FEV_1$ is less than 80% of the predicted or of their own best previously recorded values, should be tested with a

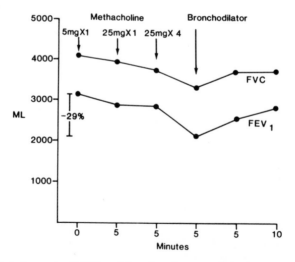

**Fig. 7-1.**   Forced vital capacity (FVC) and forced expiratory volume in one second ($FEV_1$) before (0 minutes) and following successive inhalations of methacholine at 5 mg/ml and then 25 mg/ml concentrations. Following the final four inhalations at 25 mg/ml there is a 29% fall in $FEV_1$, which is reversed with inhaled isoproterenol.

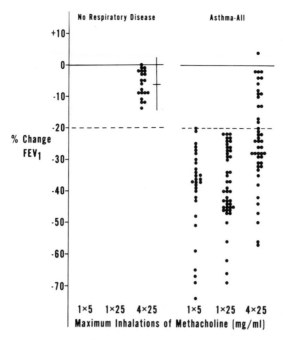

**Fig. 7-2.**    All of the patients in this study had baseline one second forced expiratory volume ($FEV_1$) greater than 80% of predicted or best previously recorded and more than 1.5 liters. Most of the asthmatic patients had a greater than 20% fall in $FEV_1$. None of the normal subjects had a fall in $FEV_1$ greater than 16%.

bronchodilator rather than methacholine if the diagnosis of asthma is in doubt. Any bronchospasm induced by methacholine should be promptly reversed to prevent development of a progressive worsening of the patient's asthma. Only rarely does a late asthmatic response follow the initial response to methacholine.

The quantitative methacholine challenge was devised to allow the safe challenge of known asthmatic patients in research studies of the natural course of the disease or the response to therapy. In this test, five metered inhalations of each concentration (0.075–25.0 mg/ml) are given. We can then construct a dose-response curve that allows us to calculate the dose that produces a 20% fall in $FEV_1$ ($PD_{20}$ $FEV_1$). Details of this method appear in Chai et al.[1]

## EXERCISE CHALLENGE

The $FEV_1$ falls significantly after certain types of exercise in more than 70% of asthmatic children. Exercise-induced bronchospasm is also a serious problem in adults. The degree of bronchospasm depends on the type and the intensity of the exercise. Running is the most asthmagenic exercise, bicycling is less so, and swimming causes the least amount of difficulty. Characteristically, bronchodilation occurs about 4 minutes after exercise begins and is then followed by bronchoconstriction. The most profound drop in $FEV_1$ occurs about 5 minutes after the exercise has ceased. The bronchospastic response is enhanced by cold, dry air and lessened by warm, humidified air.

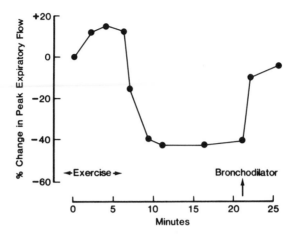

**Fig. 7-3.**   Percent change from baseline (0 minutes) expiratory flow rate during and following treadmill exercise by an adult asthmatic patient.

Figure 7-3 shows the result of exercise challenge in an individual susceptible to exercise-provoked bronchospasm.

Like methacholine challenge, exercise challenge is used both to confirm the diagnosis and to assess the response to therapy. The results of such a challenge can also be helpful in advising the asthmatic patient about exercise and athletic activities.

Prior to the test, spirometry should indicate a value greater than 80% of the individual's predicted or best previously recorded value. Patients with both asthma and ischemic heart disease (or another cardiovascular or musculoskeletal condition that may be aggravated by exercise) are sometimes not good candidates for the exercise challenge. Exercise electrocardiograph testing should precede exercise bronchospasm tests in adults known or suspected of having ischemic heart disease.

A motor-driven treadmill is most appropriate for evaluation of exercise-induced asthma. The level of stress used is determined by the patient's age, size, and degree of physical fitness. Ordinarily, bronchospasm is provoked by 5–8 minutes of steady-state exercise to 90% of predicted maximum values. The exercise begins with walking, and the rate and inclination of the treadmill are increased at 2-minute intervals until the target level of exercise is reached. The stages should not be advanced if there are cardiovascular or pulmonary signs and symptoms. The ECG is monitored continuously throughout the test. Duplicate spirometric measurements are made immediately after the exercise and at 5-minute intervals thereafter. Exercise-induced bronchospasm usually subsides within 30 minutes but can progress to a severe attack, and any patient who does not improve spontaneously should be treated with isoetharine or another bronchodilator. Details of the methodology are reported by Eggleston.[2]

## AEROALLERGEN BRONCHIAL CHALLENGE

An asthmatic patient whose disease is aggravated by an immediate hypersensitivity reaction to aeroallergen exposure usually recognizes the substance that elicits the reaction. Cat dander-sensitive individuals, for example, can often detect the presence of cats in

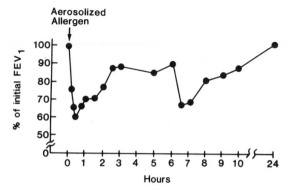

**Fig. 7-4.** Percent of baseline (0 hours) one-second forced expiratory volume ($FEV_1$) following inhalations of aerosolized antigen (method detailed in reference 1) in a sensitive asthmatic patient. An "immediate" response occurs over the first 5–30 minutes; a "late" response follows 6-8 hours later in the untreated patient.

households they are visiting by their characteristic reaction of nasal-ocular itching and watering and asthmatic symptoms that begin within 10–20 minutes after they enter the house.

The presence of IgE antibody to the putative aeroallergens in such patients may usually be confirmed by either direct prick or intradermal cutaneous tests or by tests of serum with the radioallergosorbent test (RAST) (Chapter 5). In most instances, the history or cutaneous tests will provide a sufficient basis to advise either avoidance of the aeroallergen or immunotherapy. On occasion, however, the relationship between occupational or other exposure to an aeroallergen and asthma must be confirmed by an inhalation test.

Figure 7-4 shows typical immediate and late responses to inhalations of an aeroallergen. Figure 7-5 shows how pretreatment with cromolyn sodium (Intal

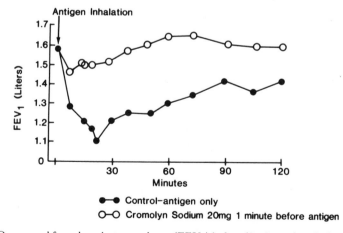

**Fig. 7-5.** One second forced expiratory volume ($FEV_1$) before (0 minutes) and after inhalations of aeroallergen on two different days in the same patient without and with pretreatment with inhalations of cromolyn. Cromolyn blocks the "immediate" and "late" (not shown) responses to aeroallergen inhalation in the sensitive asthmatic patient.

### Table 7-1
### Aeroallergen Inhalation Challenge: Limitations as Test for Clinical Relevance
### of Immediate Hypersensitivity to Asthma

| History of Asthma | Cutaneous Tests | Inhalation Test | Allergen of Importance |
|---|---|---|---|
| Positive | + | N/A (>95% +) | Yes |
| Equivocal or Negative | 0 | N/A (>95% 0) | No |
| Equivocal or Negative | + | + (~50% "false") | Possible |
| Equivocal or Negative | + | 0 | No |

[Fisons Corporation, Bedford, MA]) which blocks release of mediators of immediate hypersensitivity, can protect against allergen-provoked bronchospasm.

For investigative purposes, aeroallergen challenge may be used to measure changes in bronchial reactivity following natural exposures to an aeroallergen or to judge the effectiveness of environmental control measures, immunotherapy, or pharmacologic agents. Details of the methods and applications of aeroallergen challenges may be found in Chai et al.[1] and Rosenthal et al.[3]

Table 7-1 summarizes how aeroallergen inhalation challenge can be used to test the clinical relevance of specific reaginic antibodies in an individual with asthma.

### Table 7-2
### Reported Prevalences of Sensitivity to Other Nonsteroidal Antiinflammatory Drugs in
### Aspirin-Sensitive Patients

| | Percentage of Aspirin-Sensitive Asthma Patients |
|---|---|
| Prostaglandin Synthetase Inhibitors | |
| Indomethacin (Indocin) | 100 |
| Fenoprofen (Nalfon) | 100 |
| Naproxen (Naprosyn, Anaprox) | 100 |
| Tolmetin (Tolectin) | 100 |
| Zomepirac (Zomax) | 100 |
| Ibuprofen (Motrin) | 97 |
| Mefenamic Acid (Ponstel) | 60 |
| Sulindac (Clinoril) | ? |
| Meclofenamate (Meclomen) | ? |
| Prioxicam (Feldene) | ? |
| Possible Prostaglandin Synthetase Inhibitors | |
| Phenylbutazone (Butazolidin) | 42 |
| Acetaminophen | * |
| Nonprostaglandin Synthetase Inhibitors | |
| Sodium Salicylate | 0 |
| Choline Salicylate | 0 |
| Salicylamide | 0 |
| Propoxyphene | * |

*Isolated case report.

## ORAL CHALLENGE WITH ASPIRIN

Approximately 10% of all asthmatic patients will at some time develop hypersensitivity to aspirin and other anti-inflammatory agents that share with aspirin the ability to inhibit prostaglandin synthetase. Although the mechanism of this hypersensitivity is not understood, we do know that it is not an IgE-mediated phenomenon. Frequently it does not appear until years after the onset of rhinosinusitis, nasal polyps, and bronchial asthma. Therefore, aspirin challenge should not be used as a predictor of future reactions in such patients, since a negative challenge may well be followed, months or even years later, by a severe reaction to aspirin or aspirinlike drugs.

Table 7-2 summarizes the reported prevalence of sensitivity to other nonsteroidal anti-inflammatory drugs in aspirin-sensitive asthmatic patients. There is a direct correlation between potency as a prostaglandin synthetase inhibitor and the prevalence of cross-sensitivity.

In general, it is best to advise asthmatic patients to avoid this family of drugs. However, oral challenge with aspirin or aspirinlike drugs is occasionally desirable for the asthmatic patient with a negative, unknown, or equivocal history of sensitivity to aspirin who requires one of these agents as a platelet inhibitor because of vascular disease or as an anti-inflammatory agent for musculorheumatic disease that does not respond to non-aspirin-like drugs. Details of the methodology are reported by Mathison et al.[4]

## REFERENCES

1. Chai H, Farr RS, Froehlich LA, et al: Standardization of bronchial inhalation challenge procedures. J Allergy Clin Immunol 56:323–327, 1975
2. Eggleston PA: Laboratory evaluation of exercise-induced asthma: Methodologic considerations. J Allergy Clin Immunol 64:604–608, 1979
3. Rosenthal PR: Bronchoprovocation techniques for the evaluation of asthma. J Allergy Clin Immunol 64:561–692, 1979
4. Mathison DA, Pleskow WW, Stevenson DD, et al: Aspirin and chemical sensitivities and challenges in asthmatic patients, in Spector SC (Ed.), Provocative Challenge: Bronchial, Oral, Nasal and Exercise Procedures, Vol II. Boca Raton, Press, CRC 1983, 103–113

Part 3

# Management of the Bronchospastic Disorders: Pharmacologic Interventions

# 8

ARTHUR DAWSON

# Theophylline

Theophylline and its derivatives have been in general use for the treatment of bronchospasm since the 1930s. Since the early 1970s methods for measuring the serum level of theophylline have become available in most hospitals, and this has greatly improved our ability to adjust the dose of the drug optimally and to prevent toxic effects that are very common but often unrecognized. It was formerly believed, quite erroneously, that theophylline preparations were not well absorbed when given orally, and the major uses of this class of drugs were as intravenous (IV) aminophylline and aminophylline suppositories for acute asthma. When it was given orally, theophylline was often administered in fixed-ratio combinations with ephedrine, and the side effects of the latter often prevented the use of effective doses of theophylline. In the last few years the usefulness of single-entity oral theophylline has been recognized and the pharmaceutical industry has responded vigorously to the need for the theophylline preparations that maintain uniform blood levels of the drug over the 24-hour day. As recently as 5 years ago the "detail men" emphasized the rapid absorption and rapid achievement of peak blood levels with their products, but now we hear of narrow fluctuations of the blood level even with twice-daily dose schedules. All of this no doubt represents progress and many patients, even those with quite troublesome bronchospasm, can now be kept free of symptoms with oral theophylline alone. Theophylline should be given a trial in most asthmatics requiring regular medication, but some individuals cannot tolerate the drug, even at doses giving a subtherapeutic blood level.

## MECHANISM OF ACTION

Theophylline is believed to exert its bronchodilator effect by inhibiting the enzyme phosphodiesterase, thereby reducing the degradation of cyclic AMP (cAMP). The beta-adrenergic drugs increase cAMP by stimulating receptors of the cell membrane. This may explain the synergistic effects of these two classes of bronchodilator.

## CHEMISTRY AND METABOLISM

Theophylline is a 3-methylated xanthine and thus is closely related to caffeine in its chemical structure. Aminophylline is the ethylene diamine salt of theophylline. With the exception of dyphylline, all the methylated xanthine bronchodilators in clinical use are simple salts of theophylline; therefore, all but dyphylline can be successfully measured by the standard methods of determining serum theophylline levels.

Most of the absorbed dose of theophylline is degraded by the liver to metabolites that have little pharmacologic action. About 10% of the dose is excreted unchanged in the urine.

## SERUM LEVELS OF THEOPHYLLINE

Now that the serum theophylline can be measured in most hospitals, much of the former guesswork has been removed from selecting the correct dose of the drug.

The spectrophotometric methods formerly used had the disadvantage that the patient had to abstain from taking caffeine before the test, but high-pressure liquid chromatography (HPLC), and enzyme immunoassay are not significantly affected by caffeine or by the inactive metabolites of theophylline. Neither do they detect dyphylline (marked as Luffylin [Wallace Laboratories, Cranbury, NJ], Dilor [Savage Laboratories, Missouri City, TX], and Neothylline [Lemmon Company, Sellersville, PA]); thus serious overdosage can result if the physician attempts to regulate the dose of these preparations by using serum theophylline levels.

The HPLC method is rapid, accurate, and specific but requires a specially trained technician and equipment not available in smaller hospital laboratories. The enzyme immunoassay method uses the standard immunoassay techniques available in any clinical laboratory. However, the reagents are sold in quantities sufficient to run several dozen samples; therefore, it is relatively expensive to perform the test in a laboratory that analyzes only a few specimens daily. The results obtained by the two methods are comparable.

Table 8-1 gives the approximate relationship between serum level and therapeutic response. This table is somewhat different from tabulated data usually published and has been modified on the basis of undocumented personal experience. The important point for the practitioner to remember is that serum levels are a useful guide to dosage but there is a considerable overlap between therapeutic and toxic levels. Some patients unquestionably complain of symptoms such as sleeplessness, nausea, hiccups, and diarrhea with serum levels below 5 mg/l. Conversely, some patients seem to tolerate serum levels above 20 mg/l, but it seems hazardous not to lower the dose when the serum level is reported in this range, especially in older patients with several medical problems. The metabolism of theophylline can vary in the individual from time to time. For example, a recent patient of mine seemed to be doing well with a serum level of 22, but he returned a week later with major toxic symptoms.

When adjusting the theophylline dose on the basis of serum levels in outpatients, an additional precaution must be kept in mind. Patients should be carefully questioned as to whether they have taken *all their prescribed doses* of medication during the previous 24 hours. Apart from simple forgetfulness, many patients may deliberately omit their medication on the day of their scheduled visit, feeling for some reason that this will be helpful to the physician. Others may delay scheduling return visits until their supply of medication has run low, and they may have to ration their doses for a few days, if they have not run out altogether. Still others have learned the hard way not to refill prescriptions for expensive drugs in case their physician changes the prescription, leaving them with perhaps $15 worth of useless capsules in their medicine chests.

Table 8-1

**Relationship Between Serum Theophylline Level and Therapeutic Response**

| Serum Level, mg/l | Response | Comments |
|---|---|---|
| 5 | No effect | Some patients may experience unpleasant side effects even at these serum levels |
| 5–10 | Suboptimal therapeutic level | But the above caveat applies |
| 10–15 | Optimal therapeutic level | Major side effects (e.g., cardiac arrhythmia) can occur at these serum levels |
| 15–20 | High therapeutic level | Many patients experience toxic side effects |
| 20–25 | Usual toxic level | A few patients seem to tolerate and benefit from doses that produce these levels |
| 25 | Toxic level | There is an increased risk of major cardiac arrhythmia and convulsions |

## PHARMACOKINETICS

After a single dose of theophylline, the peak blood level achieved will depend on body size, whether the drug is given orally, and on the rate and efficiency of gastrointestinal (GI) absorption. When the drug is given by continuous IV infusion or when regular oral doses are given, the final steady-state blood levels will be determined principally by the rate of elimination of the drug that can be evaluated by calculating the serum half-life.

The half-life of theophylline varies widely between individuals, with an average of 6 hours in adults (range 3–12 hours) and 3.7 hours (range 1.4–8 hours) in children. The half-life is reduced in smokers (average 4.3 hours) and is considerably prolonged in individuals with hepatic cirrhosis and congestive heart failure.

The importance of the half-life is illustrated in Figure 8-1, in which the blood levels are calculated assuming identical rates of absorption and dosage schedule for half-lives of 4 hours and 10 hours, both values well within the normal adult range. It is apparent that if

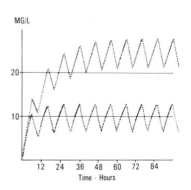

**Fig. 8-1.** Theophylline blood levels in a 70-kg man dosed with 600 mg every 12 hours, assuming absorption time of 6 hours and volume of dilution of 0.5 l/kg. The higher curve is for a half-life of 10 hours and the lower is for a half-life of 4 hours.

an optimal blood level is desired, it is useless to give a calculated dose, even on a weight basis, without monitoring the blood levels after a steady state has been achieved. Depending on the half-life and whether an initial loading dose is given, the achievement of steady state requires 12–24 hours with IV aminophylline and from 36–96 hours with theophylline tablets. From the graph shown in Figure 8-1 it is obvious that when the patient is on oral theophylline, selection of the time after the dose to sample the blood is somewhat arbitrary, but a reasonable rule is 2 hours for uncoated tablets or liquid preparations and 4–6 hours for slowly absorbed preparations.

## Pharmacologic Effects

The main therapeutic effect of theophylline is relaxation of bronchial smooth muscle, which causes bronchodilation. It also causes both systemic and pulmonary vasodilation, with the latter accounting for the fall in the arterial oxygen tension sometimes observed after IV aminophylline. It was formerly used as an effective diuretic, probably because of both renal vasodilation and a direct effect on the tubules, but this use has been superseded by the potent oral diuretics now available. It is also a central nervous system (CNS) stimulant, and in patients with depressed respiratory drive it may exert a beneficial though weak stimulant effect on the respiratory center. Occasionally this effect may be of benefit in reducing Cheyne-Stokes respirations in patients who experience distress during the hyperpneic periods. Finally, aminophylline has been shown to increase the strength of contraction and the resistance to fatigue of the diaphragm, which may be of importance in the treatment of respiratory failure.[1]

## TOXIC EFFECTS

The minor side effects of theophylline may provide a guide to when an effective dose has been achieved, but, as noted earlier, some sensitive patients will experience troublesome or even intolerable symptoms, even with "subtherapeutic" blood theophylline levels. On the other hand, serious adverse effects, even convulsions, can occur without premonitory symptoms.

Nausea is the most common side effect. Some patients will complain of nausea and epigastric burning shortly after taking the drug, in which case it is presumably due to a direct irritant effect on the gastric mucosa. Sometimes this problem can be avoided by taking the medication with food or antacid. Nausea and anorexia also occur with IV aminophylline, apparently because of both CNS and local GI effects. Less common GI problems are diarrhea and hiccups.

Patients should always be warned about the possible side effects before they begin treatment, and it is much better to be on the low side in initial dosage. Even when suitably warned, many patients lose confidence in a physician who gives them a drug that makes them sick. The natural tendency to blame such predictable adverse effects on the incompetence of the physician has been magnified by the spate of recent do-it-yourself books on therapeutics. An even more serious problem, seen much less frequently nowadays, is the patient who continues to take the medication in spite of increasing discomfort from side effects. One still occasionally encounters an ultracooperative patient who faithfully takes the theophylline or digoxin on schedule and says, "I haven't kept a thing on my stomach for 10 days."

Irritability and insomnia are common side effects of theophylline, although in the past they usually have been attributed to the sympathomimetic agents commonly prescribed with it. Tremulousness and headache are also seen frequently with toxic doses, and major convulsions can occur, usually with blood levels above 40 mg/l. Even lower blood levels than this can decrease the seizure threshold in patients predisposed to convulsions.

Cardiac arrhythmias of many types frequently occur with theophylline overdosage. Their significance may be difficult to assess in patients with chronic lung disease, however, particularly those with hypoxemia or coexisting heart disease, or those receiving several different medications likely to stimulate the heart. In general, it is desirable in patients with troublesome arrhythmias to aim for serum theophylline levels in the 10–15-mg/l range or even slightly lower before deciding to administer long-term antiarrhythmic therapy.

It must be stressed that toxicity may appear from a previously well tolerated dose of theophylline if there is any acute problem that alters the metabolic clearance of the drug. Such problems can occur during an acute respiratory infection and may be even more extreme with the development of acute hepatocellular disease or congestive heart failure.

## DRUG INTERACTIONS

Tobacco increases hepatic microsomal enzymes, thereby increasing the metabolic clearance of theophylline. This observation seems to have caught the fancy of house officers, and it is common practice to increase the initial maintenance dose of theophylline by 50% in smokers. Toxic effects frequently result. Similar effects have been attributed to the consumption of phenobarbital, marijuana, and charcoal-broiled beef, but the clinical importance of these interactions has not been established.

The metabolic clearance of theophylline has clearly been shown to be slowed by the macrolide antibiotic, troleandomycin, a fact that has become significant because of the corticosteroid-sparing effect of this agent. When troleandomycin is added in a regimen containing theophylline, the dose of the latter should be decreased by 30%–50% and the serum level should be rechecked. Erythromycin is also a macrolide antibiotic, and several studies have shown that it also slows the clearance of theophylline. One recent investigation claimed that erythromycin did not affect theophylline metabolism.[2] Until more information is available, it appears prudent to assume that the combination of an acute respiratory infection and erythromycin will require a 30% decrease in the dose of theophylline.

Recent studies have demonstrated that theophylline elimination is slowed by cimetidine[3] and by propranolol.[4] The cimetidine–theophylline interaction may be of great clinical importance since the two drugs are often given together. There are few occasions when a physician would want to prescribe theophylline and a beta-adrenergic blocking agent simultaneously.

With blood levels of many drugs available and with the increasing interest of physicians in "clinical pharmacology," we can expect many more drug interactions to be described in the next few years. Obviously it would not be cost-effective to measure the blood theophylline whenever a change is made in the patient's other medications. Whenever there seems to be a change in the patient's response to an established dose of theophylline, however, the physician should question whether there is an interaction with some other prescription or over-the-counter drug.

## INTRAVENOUS AMINOPHYLLINE

Twenty-five years ago it was a common practice to treat acute bronchospasm with aminophylline as a 500-mg bolus administered IV over 5–10 minutes. House-staff lore had it that sudden death occasionally attended such therapy, but I have never heard at first hand of any serious problem from a single dose of aminophylline given in this way, and I have certainly seen many instances of the drug's dramatic efficacy. We live in more cautious times now, and the direct injection of aminophylline into a vein can no longer be sanctioned. An initial loading dose of aminophylline is important, however, provided one is certain that *the patient has not previously been taking theophylline.* The dose should be 5–6 mg/kg (of body weight) given over 30–60 minutes, and it should be followed by maintenance therapy given by a reliable constant infusion system. The amount of this maintenance dose has been the source of much controversy. In a much quoted article, Piafsky and Ogilvie[5] recommended that the infusion be continued at 0.9 mg/kg/hr but it is now recognized that for most patients this dose is excessive.[6] Nevertheless, this figure remains enshrined in many standard references and in the little black notebooks of countless house officers. No doubt we have all had the experience of making morning rounds to find our patients who were admitted from the emergency room the previous evening relieved of their wheezes but tremulous and sleep-deprived with untasted breakfast trays at their bedsides.

More recent experience has led to the recommendations given in Table 8-2, which are for initial treatment only. The serum theophylline should be checked 12–24 hours later so that the dose can be appropriately adjusted.

## MAINTENANCE THERAPY WITH
## ORAL THEOPHYLLINE

For patients with mild asthma whose attacks occur infrequently, the use of occasional doses of oral theophylline as needed may be reasonable therapy. In such patients rapid absorption and the rapid achievement of peak blood levels is the aim of therapy. This is best accomplished by administration of plain uncoated aminophylline tablets, or, especially in children, a liquid theophylline or aminophylline preparation.

Most patients with persistent bronchospasm will benefit from oral maintenance theophylline treatment. For these patients, the aim of therapy is to provide a therapeutic blood level through the entire 24-hour day while minimizing the peaks of blood level that cause toxic side effects and the valleys that permit recurrent symptoms. Therefore, the ideal formulation is one that is slowly but efficiently absorbed over a period of 8–12 hours,

**Table 8-2**
**Recommendations for IV Aminophylline Infusion**

| | |
|---|---|
| Loading dose | 5–6 mg/kg |
| Initial maintenance dose | |
| Children 1–9 yr | 0.8 mg/kg/hr |
| Children >9 yr | 0.6 mg/kg/hr |
| Adults | 0.5 mg/kg/hr |
| Congestive heart failure or liver dysfunction | 0.2 mg/kg/hr |

preferably at a constant rate. Since the need for such preparations has been recognized, the pharmaceutical industry has responded with a host of new long-acting products. Although documentation by independent investigators of the manufacturer's claims for these preparations remains limited, there is no doubt that several products now available on the market come close to fulfilling the above requirements. It should be possible to provide satisfactory maintenance treatment for most patients with 2 or 3 doses per day.

The doses of oral theophylline currently recommended will predictably cause gastrointestinal toxicity in 10% or more of patients. As noted earlier, it usually is preferable to undershoot the starting dose and build up to an effective dose, even if it does create some delay in reaching an optimal level.

For initial therapy in an adult, it is reasonable to give approximately 200 mg every 12 hours or 150 mg every 8 hours of a long-acting preparation. If this is tolerated without side effects, the dose should be increased to 600 mg per day after 3 days. Patients can be instructed to do this themselves so that when they return a week after starting therapy, the blood level of theophylline can be checked. Thereafter, if there are no side effects, the dose can be adjusted in order to achieve the ideal level of about 15 mg/ml. Usually this can be accomplished with one or, at the most, two measurements.

Older patients or those with a history of intolerance to medications should be started on a lower test dose of 100 mg twice daily or even less. The drug should be taken with food in order to diminish local gastric irritation. It is wise to provide patients with samples or small initial prescriptions so that they will not be left with a large unused supply if they cannot tolerate the drug. The toxic symptoms themselves are soon forgotten, but the unfinished bottles remain in the medicine chests to rekindle the patients' resentment whenever they reach for fresh razor blades.

Theophylline preparations differ in their rate and efficiency of absorption, so that once the patients have gone to the trouble and expense of establishing the optimal dose, it is important that they do not switch to another brand. They may have to be reminded that in this case, as in so many others, the generic "equivalent" is not equivalent and prescriptions should be written "Do not substitute."

## OTHER THEOPHYLLINE PREPARATIONS

Recommendations for dosage are for anhydrous theophylline. If other theophylline salts are used, the dose should be adjusted according to the schedule shown in Table 8-3.

Dyphylline is in a different category because it is not a theophylline salt and the equivalent dose is unknown. Since there is no readily available blood test for dyphylline, its

**Table 8-3**
**Relative Potency of Theophylline Salts**

| Preparation | Relative Content of Theophylline | mg Equivalent to 100 mg of Anhydrous Theophylline |
|---|---|---|
| Anhydrous theophylline | 100 | 100 |
| Aminophylline | 85 | 118 |
| Oxtriphylline (Choledyl) | 64 | 155 |
| Theophylline calcium salicylate | 48 | 210 |
| Theophylline sodium glycinate | 50 | 200 |

use would no longer seem justified, except that occasional patients seem to tolerate this agent when they cannot use any oral theophylline preparation. If it is used, the dose must be established empirically. The recommended doses probably give suboptimal blood levels, which may account in part for the lower incidence of side effects.

## COMBINATION ORAL PREPARATIONS

Fixed-ratio combinations of theophylline with ephedrine can rarely be justified for modern therapy. The side effects of the ephedrine often prevent the administration of a therapeutic dose of theophylline, and the small doses of sedative added to some of the combinations are both ineffective and irrational. The synergistic effects of theophylline and ephedrine are unquestionable, but when optimal therapy is desired, it is generally preferable to prescribe one of the newer selective sympathomimetic agents—terbutaline, albuterol, or metaproterenol—and to titrate the dose. It is true that these agents are more expensive than the older combination drugs, but considering that a small fraction of the cost of health care is made up of the cost of medications, it seems false economy to skimp on the price of a drug that is demonstrably superior. Nevertheless, it is both unnecessary and poor psychology to switch a patient who is doing well on an established regimen that includes one of the combination preparations. It is likely that most of the older formulations will disappear from the market as physicians increasingly turn away from polypharmacy.

## RECTAL ADMINISTRATION

Formerly the rectal route of administration was much favored for aminophylline and theophylline, probably because of an incorrect impression that the drug was not reliably absorbed when given orally. Although aminophylline suppositories have little to recommend them because of their inconsistent absorption, occasional patients who cannot tolerate oral preparations do respond well to them. Aminophylline suppositories were formerly much used in children but may produce serious and even fatal toxicity. An especially hazardous practice that should never be used in children and should be avoided in adults is cutting suppositories in half in order to get a half-dose. Since the drug is not uniformly dispersed in the suppository, the results are unpredictable.

Rectal solutions of theophylline and aminophylline are better absorbed than suppositories and may be useful in a few patients who cannot tolerate oral theophylline but respond well to IV therapy. Both suppositories and solutions are inclined to cause local irritation if used regularly and thus they cannot be recommended for maintenance treatment.

## WHEN SHOULD THEOPHYLLINE BE USED?

For a few asthmatics with occasional brief attacks of wheezing, the symptomatic use of an inhaled sympathomimetic agent may be all that is required. For almost all others, oral therapy is indicated, and in this country theophylline is generally preferred to a sympathomimetic agent for initial treatment, although there is insufficient information to make a strong recommendation on this point.

Patients who require regular treatment and who tolerate theophylline should be given this drug in a therapeutic dose before other oral agents are added. If this does not completely control symptoms, there is both theoretical and experimental justification for using a sympathomimetic agent in addition to the theophylline, although the risk of added side effects should be recognized. It does not make sense to add a sympathomimetic to a subtherapeutic dose of theophylline unless it has been clearly shown that the patient cannot tolerate therapeutic blood levels.

When the patient requires maintenance glucocorticoid treatment, the question arises as to whether theophylline adds anything useful to the regimen. It has long been presumed by most specialists that the patient should be given the maximum tolerated doses of theophylline when an attempt is made to taper the corticosteroid dose in the hope of permitting the minimum long-term maintenance dose of the latter. This intuitive approach has recently received some support from the demonstration that theophylline produces additional bronchodilation in children on maintenance corticosteroid therapy[7] and even in patients on high-dose parenteral glucocorticoids for acute bronchospasm.

## REFERENCES

1. Aubier M, De Troyer A, Sampson M, et al: Aminophylline improves diaphragmatic contractility. New Engl J Med 305:249–252, 1981
2. Maddux MS, Leeds NH, Organek HW, et al: The effect of erythromycin on theophylline kinetics at steady state. Chest 81:563–565, 1982
3. Jackson JE, Powell JR, Wandell M, et al: Cimetidine decreases theophylline clearance. Am Rev Respir Dis 123:615–617, 1981
4. Conrad KA, Nyman DW: Effects of metoprolol and propranolol on theophylline elimination. Clin Pharmacol Ther 28:473–477, 1980
5. Piafsky KM, Ogilvie RI: Dosage of theophylline in bronchial asthma. New Engl J Med 292:1218–1222, 1975
6. Hendeles L, Weinberg M: Guidelines for avoiding theophylline overdose. New Engl J Med 300:1217, 1979
7. Nassif EG, Weinberger M, Thompson R, et al: The value of maintenance theophylline in steroid-dependent asthma. New Engl J Med 304:71–75, 1981

## SUGGESTED READINGS

Van Dallen RG: Theophylline: Practical application of new knowledge. Mayo Clin Proc 54:733–745, 1979
*Up-to-date and readable description of theophylline pharmacology.*
Ziment I: Phosphodiesterase inhibitors, Respiratory Pharmacology and Therapeutics. Philadelphia, Saunders, 1978, Chapter 6
*An outstanding chapter in an excellent book. Strongly recommended for a detailed exposition of practical aspects of theophylline prescribing.*

# 9

LAWRENCE E. KLINE

# Sympathomimetic Agents

Sympathomimetic bronchodilators are a group of drugs related to the natural catecholamines that stimulate the adrenergic receptors of the bronchial smooth muscle. Some of the practical aspects of their use in asthma are discussed in this chapter.

There are a number of sympathomimetic drugs available, and the current literature provides little guidance to the clinician as to which drug to use in what circumstances.[1] Obviously the ideal goal is to achieve the most bronchodilation for the longest possible time, with the least adverse effects. The optimal use of these agents requires careful clinical assessment supplemented by objective measures, such as spirometry.

## MECHANISM OF ACTION

The sympathomimetic agents produce bronchodilatation through the relaxation of bronchial smooth muscle. Other effects are pulmonary vasodilatation and some degree of central nervous system (CNS) stimulation. Dilatation of blood vessels in poorly ventilated regions of the lungs accounts for the hypoxemia that sometimes develops after these agents are given.

A number of additional actions occur in other parts of the body. Ahlquist[2] and Lands et al.[3] explained these various actions by their theory that there are three distinct types of adrenergic receptor now designated alpha, beta-one and beta-two receptors (Table 9-1).

Alpha agonists stimulate constriction of the smooth muscle located in arteries, veins, gastrointestinal (GI) tract sphincters, and urinary bladder trigone sphincters and possibly also in the bronchial smooth muscle. Alpha stimulation may also enhance histamine release. Most of these effects are undesirable when the drugs are given for their bronchodilator effect. Urinary retention in males, especially in the presence of prostatic hypertrophy, is an important adverse effect of drugs that produce alpha stimulation. A possibly desirable effect of the alpha agonists is mucosal vasoconstriction, which may prolong bronchodilator action and reduce mucosal engorgement. Alpha effects can be especially troublesome when bronchospasm is provoked by a beta blocker such as propranolol. The alpha adrenergic effect potentiates the beta blockade, thus bronchospasm is augmented.[4] Most of the new beta selective bronchodilators cause little alpha stimulation.

Beta adrenergic drugs stimulate cell membrane receptors, thereby increasing certain intracellular mediators. Beta receptors are divided into two categories, beta-two and

**Table 9-1**
**Major Action of Adrenergic Receptors**

| | |
|---|---|
| ALPHA | Smooth-Muscle Constriction |
| BETA-1 | Cardiac Stimulation |
| BETA-2 | Bronchodilation |
| | (Skeletal-Muscle Tremor; CNS Stimulation) |

beta-one. Beta-two receptor stimulation produces bronchodilatation, which is the desired effect. Skeletal-muscle tremor and CNS stimulation also occur when these receptors are activated. Beta-one stimulation activates cardiac receptors, increasing the heart rate and sometimes provoking ectopic beats. Fewer unwanted side effects occur with the more selective beta-two agonists. This is especially true if these agents are given by inhalation rather than by the oral or parenteral routes.

## ADVERSE EFFECTS

The adverse effects of the sympathomimetic bronchodilators are the major factor limiting their usefulness. Careful instruction to the patient prior to initiating treatment can help in achieving optimal therapy.

Urinary tract obstructive symptoms may still occur with the beta-selective drugs in the elderly male with prostatic hypertrophy, but this is a problem mainly with drugs such as ephedrine with significant alpha-stimulant action.

Tremor is a common side effect of the beta-selective bronchodilators, especially when they are given by mouth. It is most troublesome in elderly patients who may also complain of agitation, irritability, tremulousness, headache, dizziness, sweating, and insomnia. The problem is reduced if the patient is warned in advance about these side effects and if it is explained that tolerance is likely to develop in 3–4 weeks. It may help also to start with only 25–50% of the recommended maintenance dose and to increase the amount at weekly intervals. If significant side effects occur after the dose is increased, the dose should not be raised further until some degree of tolerance develops. Too rapid an increase in dose or starting therapy with the amount suggested in the current package inserts will result in many unhappy patients.

Cardiac side effects are usually due to the increased heart rate and ectopic beats associated with beta stimulation. Significant cardiac arrhythmias can occur with or without the complaint of palpitations. It may be difficult to decide whether medications are responsible for a cardiac arrhythmia since underlying heart disease, hypoxemia, acid-base disturbances, electrolyte imbalance, and other medications may be contributing factors. It is desirable to rule out and, if possible, correct other factors before reducing or discontinuing bronchodilator therapy.

The sympathomimetic bronchodilators may interact adversely with a variety of other drugs. An increased degree of stimulation can occur with monoamine oxidase (MAO) inhibitors, tricyclic antidepressants, theophylline, thyroid preparations, and antihistamines. Their use with digitalis and halogenated anesthetics may result in cardiac arrhythmias. In diabetics a rise in the blood glucose may necessitate an increase in the dose of insulin or oral hypoglycemics.

## PRINCIPLES OF TREATMENT

A beta-two selective bronchodilator can be the sole agent in a mild asthmatic with infrequent attacks. The metered dose inhaler is the ideal means of administration if it is used correctly and if it is not taken excessively. A hand-held nebulizer is equally effective, although slightly less convenient, for some patients. Some of the sympathomimetic drugs can also be given orally, but they tend to cause more systemic side effects by this route. We advise patients to use the bronchodilator at the earliest sign of an attack and prior to activities that may produce bronchospasm. This is especially helpful in patients with exercise-aggravated asthma.

In patients who require maintenance therapy for their asthma, we generally select a long-acting oral theophylline preparation in preference to an oral sympathomimetic, but some specialists prefer the latter, especially for younger individuals. When an oral theophylline preparation given in a dose sufficient to provide therapeutic blood levels does not control bronchospasm, a beta-selective bronchodilator should be added. The oral agents are convenient, for maintenance therapy, but side effects frequently limit their usefulness. Since inhaled preparations are often effective with a lower dose, it is usually preferable to administer sympathomimetics by inhalation in order to minimize systemic side effects. Because sympathomimetics and theophylline produce bronchodilatation by different but synergistic mechanisms, it is often advantageous to use them together, adjusting the dose of each independently in order to achieve the best balance between therapeutic effect and side effects. The severe asthmatic may require corticosteroids in addition, but it is still desirable to maintain the combination of a beta-selective bronchodilator and a theophylline preparation. Fixed-ratio combinations of sympathomimetic bronchodilators and theophylline are rarely justified.

The optimal dose of theophylline can be established by measuring the blood level. With sympathomimetic agents a more empirical approach is necessary. It may be sufficient to evaluate the patient's subjective response and any change in the physical findings but spirometry is an invaluable objective means of determining the results of treatment. If the purpose of the spirometry is to assess patient response to therapy, it is important to advise the patient not to discontinue medication prior to the test, as pulmonary function laboratories sometimes recommend. Serial spirometry may be especially helpful as a means of detecting a decline in lung function in a patient whose medications are being reduced and may detect a significant change before there is any clinical deterioration. Home monitering of peak flow rate can successfully detect an early decline in lung function. A pattern of fluctuating peak flow rates throughout the day or "morning dipping" with little airways obstruction during the daytime can alert the patient and clinician to a need for more vigorous therapy.[5,6]

## ADMINISTRATION OF THE DRUG

Inhaled bronchodilators can be given by a hand-bulb or pressurized nebulizer, an intermittent positive-pressure breathing device, or a metered-dose inhaler. In the first two methods the volume of diluent, the volume of the medication, and the time of administration or the number of inhalations are prescribed. The metered dose inhaler is prescribed by the number of puffs. The depth a metered cannister sinks in a container of water is directly

**Table 9-2**
**Cleaning the Metered Dose Inhaler**

1. Clean mouthpiece and cap in liquid detergent and rinse with hot running water.

2. Soak in 1/4 cup water and equal quantity of white vinegar for 30 minutes.

3. Dry with towel.

4. Rinse tip of dispenser in hot running water.

proportional to the approximate drug volume. If the cannister sinks to the bottom it is full, approximately 200 puffs, and if it floats to the top it is empty. The approximate number of remaining puffs can be estimated by this technique.

The potential advantage of the aerosol technique in minimizing systemic side effects is limited by the amount of medication deposited in the orpharynx and absorbed systemically, which may be as much as 90% or more of the nebulized drug. Aerosol therapy can also be irritating to the tracheobronchial tree. Absorption through the oral mucosa is reduced if patients rinse their mouths after each treatment. The patient's technique should be carefully checked initially and reviewed periodically to assure maximal inhalation of available medication. Details of the technique of using a metered dose inhaler are given in Chapter 4. The device must be cleaned daily (Table 9-2). The mouthpiece and cap can be cleaned with liquid detergent and rinsed under hot running water and then should be soaked in a solution of one-quarter cup of water and an equal amount of white vinegar for 30 minutes. This helps to keep the device clean and, most importantly, helps keep the jet opening clear. After soaking, the plastic mouthpiece should be dried with a towel. The tip of the dispenser should also be rinsed under hot running water daily to keep the tip and its small pinhole free from a buildup of medication.

A valved holding chamber has been developed to overcome the problem experienced by some patients in coordinating their inspiration with activation of the inhaler. This device is an 11 × 4-m rigid plastic cylinder called an *aerochamber*.[7,8] It has an adapter for the metered spray on one end and a valved mouthpiece on the other. The valve prevents exhalation into the chamber and allows inhalation of the aerosol once it is discharged into the chamber.

Oral or parenteral therapy may be necessary when adequate aerosol delivery to diseases lung sites cannot be achieved. This may also be the preferred means of administration in patients who tend to abuse inhaled medications.

## CHOOSING A DRUG

One should try to select the most effective and best tolerated sympathomimetic bronchodilator. This translates into maximal bronchodilation (beta-two-effect), minimal cardiac stimulation (beta-one effect), and long duration of action with the least side effects. Since not all the currently available drugs are available in aerosol, metered-dose inhaler, and oral and parenteral forms, the desired route of administration will also limit the choice of agents. In general, aerosolized drugs give the greatest amount of bronchodilatation with the least troublesome side effects, but oral agents should be used when there is some reason to avoid the inhaled route of administration. For example, in some patients aerosol sprays of any type are simply too irritating, and some cannot use an inhaler adequately. The convenience of taking a pill may be appealing enough to some patients to improve compliance.

Injection is the best way to give a sympathomimetic during an acute exacerbation when a reliable immediate effect is needed, but it must be used with caution, if at all, in patients over 40 years of age with heart disease or hypertension. Injections are rarely desirable for maintenance treatment in the patient with chronic asthma.

## SPECIFIC SYMPATHOMIMETIC DRUGS

### Nonselective Drugs

The available sympathomimetic bronchodilators are considered according to their degree of beta-two selective action. Ephedrine and epinephrine are not selective agents. They have alpha, beta-two and beta-one actions.

#### Epinephrine

Epinephrine is a natural catecholamine that has been used for many years. It is generally given subcutaneously as the initial therapy in young asthmatics. Adverse effects include palpitations, tachyarrhythmias, headache, agitation, diaphoresis, angina pectoris, hypertension, urinary retention, and CNS stimulation. The aerosol form is widely available as both an over-the-counter and a prescription preparation.

When bronchospasm is provoked by beta blockers, epinephrine may worsen the condition. This is because the combination of the alpha-adrenergic effect of the epinephrine with the beta blockade potentiates the bronchospastic mechanism.[9]

#### Ephedrine

Ephedrine is the active ingredient in the herb *ma huang*, which has been used by the Chinese to treat asthma for over 5000 years. It is not a catecholamine, but it stimulates the release of endogenous catecholamines from storage granules. Like epinephrine, it has alpha, beta-two, and a marked beta-one action. Ephedrine is well absorbed when given orally and has a plasma half-life of 3–12 hours. The onset of action is gradual over 1 hour and lasts for about 4 hours after a 25-mg oral dose.[10]

Since catecholamine storage granules must be released for ephedrine to be effective, tachyphylaxis is a common problem with its prolonged use. When it is combined with theophylline and a tranquilizer (e.g., Marax [Roerig, New York, NY], Tedral [Parke-Davis, Morris Plains, NJ]), the drug is better tolerated, but the use of such fixed-ratio combinations is undesirable because the side effects of the ephedrine often make it impossible to give the patient enough theophylline to provide a therapeutic blood level. Combination drug therapy is generally to be discouraged; however, in a few patients who are doing well on an established regimen containing one of these preparations, there is no reason to change, especially since these medications are generally cheaper than the new single-entity drugs.

Ephedrine is not a good choice for the management of asthma now that better agents are available. It is an unreliable bronchodilator that has many side effects and can cause tachyphylaxis.

## Beta Selective Therapy

Isoproterenol is the prototype beta agonist with strong beta-one and beta-two actions. Although it is beta-selective compared to ephedrine and epinephrine, in addition to the desired beta-two action it has a potent and undesirable beta-one action. It is usually given by inhalation, but oral and intravenous (IV) preparations are available. The duration of effect following aerosol administration varies from 20 to 120 minutes.

A sevenfold increase in the number of deaths from asthma was noted in the United Kingdom during the 1960s.[11] Several explanations for this problem have been suggested, but since the metered-dose spray used in England was five times as concentrated as the spray available in the United States, overdosage is the most likely cause of the increased mortality. Other proposed explanations were overuse of the aerosol and a toxic reaction to the fluorocarbon propellant, although the latter is unlikely.[9] Paradoxical bronchospasm due to the elaboration of beta blockers as metabolic products of large doses of isoproterenol has also been suggested. Bronchoconstriction after the administration of isoproterenol is rare, but instances have been documented.[12] Tachyphylaxis is another concern since tolerance can develop to both beta-one and beta-two effects. If larger and more frequent doses of the aerosol are needed, therefore, the patient should be switched to alternate forms of therapy.

The beta-one cardiostimulatory effects of isoproterenol and its short duration of action are relative disadvantages compared with the newer, more selection beta-two agents.

### Beta-two-Selective Therapy

Currently four major beta-two-selective bronchodilators are available. They vary to some degree in potency and duration of action, but they last longer than isoproterenol and cause less cardiac stimulation, although they are not quite as potent. These drugs include isoetharine, metaproterenol, terbutaline, and albuterol. Fenoterol should become available soon and promises to be even more beta-two-selective with somewhat greater potency and duration of action than the other drugs mentioned.[13]

Isoetharine has negligible alpha activity and less beta-one and beta-two activity than isoproterenol. The degree of cardiac stimulation  or beta-one action is similar to that of metaproterenol and terbutaline depending on the dose used. Albuterol and fenoterol have diminished cardiac effects in comparison with the other agents mentioned. Even so, they are not as free of beta-one effects as the commercial literature seems to indicate.

The duration of action varies with each of the beta-two selective bronchodilators (see Table 9-3). This difference can be important when deciding which drug to use. A shorter-acting agent may be used late in the day so that the unwanted side effects are less apt to interfere with sleep. However, the agent with the longest action is generally preferred.

The bronchodilator effect of the isoetharine lasts from 1 to 3 hours. The half-life decreases with intensive use and varies considerably between individuals. Metaproterenol has a somewhat longer maximal duration of action, ranging from 3 to 5 hours. Neither tachyphylaxis nor paradoxic bronchospasm has been a problem with metaproterenol. Terbutaline, an analog of metaproterenol, is effective for 4–7 hours. It is soon to be released as a metered inhaler in the United States. Albuterol, known as salbutamol outside the United States, has a similar duration of action. Albuterol is the preferred drug because it is highly beta-two-selective, the most potent, and currently the longest-acting available sympathomimetic agent available as an inhaled preparation.

**Table 9-3**
**Beta-two-Selective Sympathomimetic Drugs**

| Drug | Duration, Hours | Metered | Solution Concentration* |
|------|-----------------|---------|-------------------------|
| Isoetherarine | 1–3 | 340 μg/Puff | 0.25–1 ml, 1% solution (1 ml = 10 mg) |
| Metaproterenol | 3–5 | 650 μg/Puff | 0.1–0.3 ml 5% solution (0.2 ml = 15 mg) |
| Terbutaline | 4–7 | 250 μg/Puff† | 0.25–1.5 mg Injectable‡ |
| Albuterol | 4–6 | 90 μg/Puff | 0.1–1 mg† |
| Fenoterol | 6–8 | 200 μg/Puff† | 0.5–1 mg† |

*Dosage frequency ranges from 3 to 6 hours, depending on the duration of action. The solution dose is usually diluted in 1.5–3 ml of saline or water.
†Soon to become available in the United States.
‡The injectable form has been used in an inhaled aerosol, although it is not FDA-approved.

When fenoterol is released in the United States, it may offer significant advantages over the other drugs mentioned.[13] This agent is a derivative of metaproterenol with a duration of at least 8 hours when given either orally or by aerosol. It is also more potent and beta-two-selective; thus its cardiovascular and CNS side effects should be less.

An enlarging list of beta-two-selective sympathomimetic bronchodilators is under investigation. Some of these include salmefamol, stoerenol, ibuterol, carbuterol, clenbuterol, ritodrine, and pirbuterol. The goal of maximal beta-two selectivity and effectiveness with minimal side effects may be realized in these newer agents.

## DOSAGE

### Epinephrine, Ephedrine, and Isoproterenol

#### Epinephrine

Epinephrine is available in an injectable form as 1:1000 (0.1%) solution. The usual dose, 0.1–0.5 ml given subcutaneously, can be repeated in 30 minutes to a maximum of 1.0 mg (1 ml). This total dose can be repeated every 4–6 hours, but if repeated doses are needed, it is generally advisable to consider another drug. Susphrine is a 1:200 aqueous suspension that exerts a more prolonged effect, lasting from 8 to 10 hours. The maximum dose in adults is 0.3 ml every 4 hours and for children, not more than 0.15 ml every 8 hours. There is also a preparation of epinephrine in oil for intramuscular (IM) administration whose effect lasts up to 16 hours, but because it can cause sterile abscesses at the injection site, it should no longer be used.

The aerosol form of epinephrine is widely available in both over-the-counter and prescription preparations. A racemic mixture is available as a 2.25% solution of epinephrine for intermittent positive-pressure breathing (IPPB) or nebulizer use. The adult dose is two to six inhalations given four to six times a day by nebulizer or 0.3 to 1.0 ml diluted or undiluted every 2 to 4 hours by IPPB. With the potent beta-two selective aerosol preparations now available, it is undesirable to use epinephrine in this form. One should be alert to patients who have been abusing the over-the-counter form of this drug, which causes excessive cardiovascular and CNS stimulation with suboptimal bronchodilatation.

### Ephedrine

The dose of ephedrine in adults is 15–50 mg. four times a day. In children age 2–6 years a dose of 0.3–0.5 mg/kg daily and in older children, a dose of 6.25–12.5 mg at most every 4 hours was used. The "was" is emphasized since ephedrine is a poor choice for asthma treatment today because of the availability of more effective oral sympathomimetic agents in the past 10 years. As mentioned previously, it is unreliable in effect, has too many side effects and it results in tachyphylaxis.

### Isoproterenol

Metered isoproterenol aerosols deliver 0.04–0.125 mg per puff depending on the product used. A smaller dose, as low as 0.02 mg, can yield a maximal response in some patients.[14] The dose is one to four puffs every 4–6 hours. A dilution of 0.5 ml of a 1:200 solution of isoproterenol mixed with 2 ml of water or normal saline can be administered by IPPB or nebulizer (hand-bulb or compressor). The beta-one cardiostimulatory effects of this drug and its short duration of action are disadvantages not present in the newer more selective beta-two agents.

Oral or sublingual doses of 5–30 mg every 4–6 hours and IV therapy of 0.1 $\mu$g/kg/min were occasionally used in the past to treat bronchospasm, but these forms have been superseded in recent years by the new beta-two selective agents.

### Isoetharine

The metered-dose preparation contains 340 $\mu$g/puff. A dose of 1–4 puffs every 3–6 hours, with a maximum of 12 puffs/day, is the usual therapeutic range (see Table 9-2). When used by IPPB or nebulizer, approximately 0.25–0.5 ml can be diluted with 1.5–3.0 ml of water or saline. A maximum of 1.0 ml of the drug can be used if necessary. No oral preparation of this agent is available in the United States.

### Metaproterenol

The metered-dose aerosol delivers 640 $\mu$g/puff as a micronized powder. A dose of one to three puffs every 3–4 hours with a maximum of 12 puffs per day is recommended. A 5% solution for use with IPPB or nebulizers has been released recently. The manufacturer recommends a dilution of 0.3 ml mixed with a 2.5 ml of water or saline (see Table 9-3). When a hand nebulizer is used, 5–15 inhalations of the undiluted solution can be given. This is a very concentrated solution, with 15 mg in each 0.3-ml dose. Wider usage and better comparative studies will help to determine whether the side effects become a limiting factor. We find that a dose of 0.1–0.15 ml is better tolerated than the recommended dose. However, some patients complain of excessive sympathomimetic stimulation even with this smaller amount.

The oral preparation is available as a syrup and as tablets (see Table 9-4). In adults a dose of 10–20 mg three to four times a day is recommended. More sympathomimetic side effects, such as tremor and tachycardia, are experienced with this form. As with isoproterenol, IV use is not recommended.

### Terbutaline

When given orally, terbutaline is a very effective bronchodilator but it is often poorly accepted by patients because of the harmless but very unpleasant side effect of muscle tremor. The manufacturer's literature recommends that terbutaline be given orally in a dose of 2.5–5 mg three or four times daily (see Table 9-4). In order to minimize muscle tremor, it is advisable to start at a low dose (1.25 mg twice a day) and gradually to increase it to maximum over the first 2–3 weeks of therapy. The parenteral form is given in a dose of 0.125–0.25 mg subcutaneously, which can be repeated in 30 minutes. No more than 0.5 mg should be given during a 4-hour period. Theoretically, terbutaline should cause less tachycardia than epinephrine when it is given parenterally, but a recent clinical study showed that tachycardia was greater for terbutaline compared to epinephrine for the same degree of bronchodilatation.[5] In patients with congestive heart failure, terbutaline can improve left ventricular function,[6] which might be a reason for its cautious use in the asthmatic with congestive heart failure.

The aerosol form is not available in this country, but some specialists have prepared an aerosol from the injectable solution (see Table 9-3). A dose of 0.25–1.5 mg can be diluted with an equal volume of water or saline and administered by IPPB or nebulizer. Up to 1.5 mg has been used by this method at one time without significant side effects.[7] A maximum of 2.0 mg/day should be effective. A metered aerosol, will be available soon in the United States and delivers 0.250–0.375 mg/puff. The recommended dose is one to four puffs three or four times per day.

### Albuterol and Fenoterol

The aerosol form of albuterol and fenoterol is very similar to terbulaline[18] (see Table 9-3). Albuterol is now available in the United States as both a metered-dose inhaler and as tablets. The metered-dose pressurized aerosol provides 0.09 mg with each inhalation. It may take up to an hour after inhalation for albuterol to show its peak effect, a slower onset of action than that of either isoproterenol or metaproterenol, which are effective 5–6 minutes after inhalation. The recommended dose of the metered aerosol is two puffs (0.18 mg) every 4–6 hours.

The oral form (see Table 9-4) of albuterol is slightly more potent than terbutaline and has similar sympathomimetic side effects, especially tremor.[19] The oral dose is 4 mg four times a day but can be reduced if necessary. As with terbutaline, it is preferable to start with 1 mg twice a day and to gradually increase the dose over 2–3 weeks. Although albuterol causes less cardiac stimulation than terbutaline, tremor is a persistent problem. When albuterol is delivered by nebulizer or IPPB, 2 ml of a 0.5% solution provides 10 mg. Albuterol can also be administered IV at a rate of 4 $\mu$g/min or 0.05–0.2 $\mu$g/kg/min. Neither the 0.5% solution nor the IV preparation is currently available in the United States.

Fenoterol should soon be available in the United States. It appears very promising and may become the sympathomimetic agent of choice. An aerosol dose of 0.4 mg every 8 hours or an oral dose of 7.5 mg every 8–12 hours is recommended[20,21] (see Tables 9-3 and 9-4).

**Table 9-4**
**Oral Beta-Two Selective Sympathomimetic Drugs**

| Drug | Tab, mg | Adult Dose, mg |
|------|---------|----------------|
| Metaproterenol | 10, 20 | 10–20 q6h |
| Albuterol | 2, 4 | 2–4 q6h |
| Terbutaline | 2.5, 5 | 1.25–5 q6–8h |
| Fenoterol | 7.5* | 7.5 q8–12h |

*Not available in the United States.

## CONCLUSION

This survey of sympathomimetic agents is intended as a source of practical information for the clinician. Several reviews have been published that the reader should consult for details of chemical structure, mechanism of action, and pharmacokinetics.[22-25]

## REFERENCES

1. Ziment I: Pharmacology of sympathomimetic agents, in Respiratory Pharmacology and Therapeutics. Philadelphia, Saunders 1978, p 147
2. Ahlquist RP: A study of the adrenotropic receptors. Am J Physiol 153:586–600, 1948
3. Lands AM, Arnold M: Differentiation of receptor systems activated by sympathomimetic amines. Nature 214:597–598, 1967
4. Ziment I: Pharmacology of sympathomimetic agents, in Respiratory Pharmacology and Therapeutics, Philadelphia, Saunders, 1978, p 171
5. Turner-Warwick, M: On Observing Patterns Of Airflow Obstruction In Chronic Asthma. Br J Dis Chest 71:73, 1977
6. Turner-Warwick, M: Some Clinical Problems in Patients with Airways Obstruction Chest 82:35, 1982 (suppl)
7. Corr D, Dolovich M, McCormack D, et al: Design and characteristics of a portable breath actuated, particle size selective medical aerosol inhaler. J Aerosol Sci 13:1–7, 1982
8. Corr D, Dolovich M, McCormack D, et al: The aerochamber: A new demand-inhalation device for delivery of aerosolized drugs. Am Rev Respir Dis 121 (part 2 of 2):123, 1980
9. Clark D, Tinston D: Cardiac effects of isoproterenol, hypoxia, hypercapnia, and fluorocarbon propellants and their use in asthma inhalers. Ann Allergy 30:536–641, 1972
10. Pickup MD, May C, Ssendagire R, et al: The pharmacokinetics of ephedrine after oral dosage in asthmatic receiving acute and chronic treatment. Br J Clin Pharmacol. 3:123–134, 1976
11. Stolley PD: Asthma mortality. Why the United States was spared an epidemic of deaths due to asthma. Rev Respir Dis 105:883–890, 1972
12. Van Metre RE: Adverse effects of inhalation of excessive amounts of nebulized isoproterenol in status asthmatics. J Allergy 43:101, 1969
13. Watanabe S, Turner WG, Renzetti A, et al: Bronchodilator effects of nebulized fenoterol. Chest 80:292, 1981
14. Williams MH, Kane C: Dose response of patient with asthma to inhaled isoproterenol. Am Rev Respir Dis 115:321–324, 1975
15. Sackner W, Dougherty, Watson, et al: Hemodynamic effects of epinephrine and terbutaline in normal saline. Chest 68:616, 1975
16. Slutsky R, Hooper W, Gerber K, et al: Left ventricular size and function after subcutaneous administration of terbutaline. Chest 79:501, 1981
17. Glass P, Dulfano MJ: Evaluation of a new beta-two adrenergic receptor stimulant in bronchospasm. III. Aerosol administration. Curr Ther Res 18:425–432, 1975
18. Choo-Kary YF, MacDonald H, Horne N: A comparison of salbutamol and terbutaline aerosols in bronchial asthma. Practitioner 211:801, 1973
19. Legge JS, Gaddie J, Palmer K: Comparison of two oral selective beta-two adrenergic stimulant drugs in bronchial asthma. Br Med J 1:637–639, March 1979
20. Steen SN, Smith R, Juo J, et al: Comparison of the bronchodilator effects of oral therapy with fenoterol hydrobromide and ephedrine. Chest 72:291–295, 1977
21. Steen SN, Smith R, Kuo J, et al: Comparison of the bronchodilator effects of aerosol fenterenol and isoproterenol. Chest 72:724–730, 1977

22. Paterson J, Woolcock A, Shenfield G: Bronchodilator drugs. State of the art. Am Rev Respir Dis 120:1149, 1979.

23. Van Arsdel P, Paul G: Drug therapy in the management of asthma. Ann Int Med 87:68–74, 1977

24. Webb-Johnson D, Andrews J: Bronchodilator therapy. New Engl J Med 297:476–482, 1977

25. Nelson HS: Beta adrenergic agonists. Chest 82 (suppl):338, 1982

# 10

DONALD D. STEVENSON

# Systemic Corticosteroids

Corticosteroids are hormones secreted by the adrenal cortex consisting of mineralocorticoids with renal sodium retaining functions and glucocorticoids that alter carbohydrate metabolism. The glucocorticoids have important anti-allergic and anti-inflammatory effects, and synthetic derivatives of the glucocorticoids have been developed that accentuate the therapeutic effects and diminish mineralocorticoid effects. Table 10-1 lists those corticosteroids generally used at this time for the treatment of asthma.

All corticosteroid preparations have the same potential for improving asthma. Their side effects depend on dosage, length and schedule of administration, and individual susceptibility of the patient receiving the drug.

The therapeutic effects of corticosteroids in the management of asthma are impressive. These drugs are the most important pharmocologic agents in the treatment of asthma. The possible mechanisms by which glucocorticoids exert their beneficial effects in asthma are listed in Table 10-2.

For their great therapeutic benefits, the glucocorticoids exact a heavy cost in the form of adverse effects on other tissues of the body, including decreased protein synthesis, enhancement of adiposity, and suppression of immune defenses. These side effects limit the usefulness of glucocorticoids, despite the fact that almost any degree of asthma activity can be reversed if glucocorticoids are administered early enough in sufficient doses. The purpose of the next section is to describe therapeutic strategies for using these drugs, emphasizing their short-term use. The final section discusses indications for the long-term use of corticosteroids and some strategies that can be used to minimize their adverse effects.

## SHORT-TERM USE OF GLUCOCORTICOIDS

Fortunately, it takes approximately 3–4 weeks of continuous systemic glucocorticoid therapy to suppress pituitary ACTH secretion (creating relative adrenal insufficiency) and initiate the long-term, nonreversible adverse side effects. From a practical standpoint, therefore, one can administer large doses of glucocorticoids during this 3–4-week interval and expect complete adrenal recovery at the end of treatment with no long-term adverse effects. Short-term side effects are dependent on dosage and individual susceptibility of the patient and are generally reversible. Hypertension, diabetes mellitus, obesity, psychosis, glaucoma, and esophageal reflux all predispose to greater problems with these drugs.

## Table 10-1
### Glucocorticoid Preparations

| | Potency, Unit | Equivalence, mg | IV or IM | Oral | Cost |
|---|---|---|---|---|---|
| **Short-acting** | | | | | |
| Hydrocortisone | 1.0 | 20 | Yes | Yes | Moderate |
| **Intermediate-Acting** | | | | | |
| Prednisone | 3.5 | 5 | No | Yes | Lowest |
| Prednisolone | 4.0 | 5 | No | Yes | Low |
| Methyl prednisolone | 5.0 | 4 | Yes | Yes | High |
| **Long-Acting** | | | | | |
| Triamcinolone | 10.0 | 4 | Yes | Yes | High |
| Dexamethasone | 30.0 | 0.75 | Yes | Yes | High |


## Table 10-2
### Pharmacologic Effects of Glucocortoids Relevant to Treatment of Asthma

Delays and/or partially inhibits reaccumulation of intracellular histamine after discharge

Anti-inflammatory effects
  Decreased eosinophil accumulation
  Decreased circulating lymphocytes, macrophages, and monocytes; Sequestration in reticuloendothelial system
  Impaired bacteriologic activity by polymorphonuclear leukocytes and monocytes
  Blocked prostaglandin synthesis: preventing formation of arachidonic acid.

Reverses beta-adrenergic blockade
Inhibits Phosphodiesterase activity

Increased intracellular cyclic AMP activity
  Blunts (does not inhibit) mediator release
  Increased glycogenolysis: Relaxes smooth muscle


## Table 10-3
### Short-Term Adverse Side Effects from Systemic Glucocorticoids

| Effect | Consequences | Therapy |
|---|---|---|
| Increased appetite | Weight gain | Reduce caloric intake |
| NaCl and $H_2O$ retention | Edema | Reduce NaCl intake |
| Hyperacidity | Esophagitis, gastritis | Antacids, cimetidine |
| Hypertension | Headaches, CVA | Monitor blood pressure; treat as necessary |
| Psychosis | Disruptive behavior, personal injury | Major tranquilizers |
| Increased intraocular pressure | Glaucoma (pain) | Tonometry, ophthalmology consult |
| Hypokalemia | Weakness | KCl replacement |
| Increased gluconeogenesis | Poor control, diabetes mellitus | Diet, hypoglycemic agents |

## Table 10-4
## Indications for Short-Term Treatment with Glucocorticoids in Asthma

Absolute requirement to treat
    Status asthmaticus
    Previous prolonged corticosteroid therapy now under stress, (asthma, operation)

Relative requirement to treat
    Diagnostic test—asthma vs fixed COPD
    Moderately severe asthma in relapse
      Temporary allergen exposure
      Respiratory infection
      Air pollution alert
      Aspirin-induced asthma attack

## Table 10-5
## Dosages of Glucocorticoids to Treat Status Asthmaticus*

| Preparation (IV) | Adult | | Child | |
|---|---|---|---|---|
| | Initial† | 24 Hours | Initial† | 24 Hours |
| Hydrocortisone | 200 mg | 600 mg | 3 mg/kg | 8 mg/kg |
| Methyl prednisolone | 125 mg | 245 mg | 1 mg/kg | 3 mg/kg |

*Occasional patients require larger dosages.
†Initial—IV push bolus.

## Table 10-6
## Dosages of Glucocorticoids to Prevent Adrenal Insufficiency Under Stress for 24 Hours*

| Preparation | Adult | Child |
|---|---|---|
| Hydrocortisone (IV) (IM) | 400 mg | 8 mg/kg |
| Methyl prednisolone (IV, IM) | 80 mg | 1.5 mg/kg |
| Prednisone (0) | 100 mg | 2 mg/kg |

*Surgery, asthma relapse, auto accident, etc.

## Table 10-7
## Dosages of Glucocorticoids Used to Differentiate Asthma from Fixed COPD

Baseline spirometry pre- and postbronchodilator
Prednisone (0)
    Adults—80 mg/day for 3 days
    Children—2 mg/kg/day for 3 days

Repeat spirometry pre- and postbronchodilator

## Table 10-8
## Dosages of Glucocorticoids Used to Treat Severe but Self-Limited Asthma

Prednisone (0)
    Adult—80 mg/day for 5–10 days to clear asthma
    Child—2 mg/kg/day for 5–10 days to clear asthma
    Taper over 7–21 days to 0 or alternate day schedule

Table 10-3 lists the short-term side effects produced by systemic glucocorticoids and the strategies for reducing or eliminating them.

In determining the indications for the short-term use of systemic corticosteroids, we must examine the balance between these variables: (1) severity of the asthma, (2) probability that the provoking factor for the asthma will be gone or diminished in 3–4 weeks, and (3) individual susceptibility of the patient who is about to receive corticosteroids.

Table 10-4 lists those situations where asthma absolutely must be treated with corticosteroids and those where judgment must determine whether the short-term use of corticosteroids is justified.

In the short-term use of corticosteroids, it is better to lean toward overusing these drugs as long as it appears reasonably certain that the provoking factor will clear within 1 month. The reason for this is that even in England, where universal health care is at least theoretically available, about 1500 asthmatics die of respiratory obstruction each year. In most cases, the patient is documented to have severe asthma for 2–3 weeks before death and during this time has one to five encounters with the medical profession where steroids are either withheld or used in such homeopathic dosages that the asthma is never adequately treated. Withholding corticosteroids to protect the patient from potential side effects may actually produce the ultimate adverse effect, death from asthma.

The optimal dosages of corticosteroid are unknown. However, the general principle is that once the decision to give steroids has been made, enough should be given and high dosage continued until the asthma clears. The dose is then tapered over 1–3 weeks, depending on the underlying provoking factors, how rapidly the asthma has cleared, whether there are acute side effects, and whether there is any recurrence of asthma during tapering of corticosteroids. Tables 10-5–10-8 list dosages of corticosteroids that I use in treating asthma under different conditions. However, there are no controlled studies that indicate what dosages are effective or ineffective in these clinical settings.

## LONG-TERM USE OF
## SYSTEMIC GLUCOCORTICOIDS

Virtually all chronic asthma can be controlled with daily dosages of systemic corticosteroids if that dosage is maintained at a sufficiently high level. In chronic asthma, therefore, the most serious consequence of the disease can be the side effects of the drug used to control it. This section is thus devoted to three issues:

1. How does the physician determine which chronic asthmatic needs systemic corticosteroids?
2. What are the long-term adverse effects of corticosteroids?
3. What can be done to minimize or eliminate these side effects?

## RECOGNITION OF THE ASTHMATIC
## PATIENT WHO MIGHT REQUIRE
## SYSTEMIC CORTICOSTEROIDS

Development of a profile of each new asthmatic is helpful in identifying provoking factors that might be eliminated and hence will not continue to stimulate asthma. At the same time, certain subtypes of asthma can be recognized that cannot be adequately

### Table 10-9
### Subtypes of Asthma Generally Requiring
### Long-Term Systemic Corticosteroids

Allergic pulmonary aspergillosis
Postviral (Influenza)-onset asthma
Asthmatic bronchitis in relapse
Some forms of idiopathic asthma

### Table 10-10
### Possible Determinants of Adverse Effects with Long-Term
### Corticosteroid Therapy

Patient's Biological Response to corticosteroids.
Corticosteroid Preparation Used
Dosage Needed to Control Wheezing
Dosage Schedule (qid, qd, qod)
Measures Available to Counter Side Effects
Patient Compliance

### Table 10-11
### Mild to Moderate Side Effects of Systemic Corticosteroids

Increased appetite
Edema
Facial erythema
Facial fullness
Cutaneous changes: acne, striae, ecchymosis,
   and hypertrichosis
CNS effects: insomnia, headache, mood changes
Nocturia
Leg cramps

### Table 10-12
### Serious Adverse Effects of Systemic Corticosteroids

| Side Effect | Countermeasure |
|---|---|
| Growth retardation (children) | Alternate-day prednisone |
| Muscle atrophy | Exercise |
| Poor wound healing | Meticulous wound care |
| Diabetes: Poor control | Increase insulin |
| Suppression of adrenal | Replacement during stress |
| Diminished, delayed hypersensitivity | TB surveillance Isoniazid when Indicated |
| Osteoporosis (postmenopausal) | Calcium, vitamin D, estrogen |
| Posterior subcapsular cataracts | Surgery |
| Hypokalemia | KCl Replacement |
| Decreased serum IgG | Unknown |
| Hypertension | Antihypertensive Therapy |

controlled without some treatment schedule of systemic corticosteroids. These subtypes are listed in Table 10-9 and when recognized, should be treated early with systemic corticosteroids, because chances of control without steroids are very low. A number of other subtypes of asthma may require intermittent steroids. Sometimes continued exposure to cigarette smoking or infection (e.g., chronic sinusitis) may produce what appears to be a "steroid-dependent" asthmatic. The diagnosis of reversible obstructive airways diseases must be firmly established before one considers using medications with such potential long-term adverse effects. Furthermore, if time permits, nonsteroidal medications should be used first, and only after they have proved themselves to be inadequate should corticosteroids be added.

## POTENTIAL COMPLICATIONS
## OF SYSTEMIC CORTICOSTEROIDS

In general, adverse effects from systemic cortisteroids are related to the variables listed in Table 10-10.

Adverse effects from systemic corticosteroids are variable. Some are mild, easily tolerated, and do not have long-term consequences. Others are cosmetically unacceptable (ecchymosis, striae, hypertrichosis) but will not cause other health problems. Finally, some side effects are intolerable to both the patient and the physician.

Table 10-11 lists those non-acute side effects that the patient can usually tolerate. It should be noted that weight gain and skin changes are sometimes unacceptable to certain patients. If the corticosteroids were appropriately prescribed in the beginning, however, withdrawal of the "unacceptable" corticosteroids leads to even more unacceptable asthma. Table 10-12 lists the more serious side effects.

In postmenopausal woman, corticosteroids accelerate osteoporosis and the routine use of calcium supplements (enough to provide 1000 mg/day) along with vitamin D 50,000 units/wk is desirable. Estrogen replacement in women and androgen replacement in men are also helpful. It is important to realize that many so-called adverse side effects that have been attributed to corticosteroids may be coincidental, related to the underlying disease, or secondary to another process. Peptic ulcer disease, pancreatitis, aseptic necrosis of the bone all fall into this category. The Physician's Desk Reference (PDR) lists so many "adverse effects" of corticosteroids that it has ceased to be a useful document for consultation regarding side effects.

## STRATEGIES TO COUNTER SIDE EFFECTS BY
## DRUG AND DOSAGE SCHEDULES

If systemic corticosteroid therapy is initiated in a situation where it may have to be continued for more than a month, the nonsteroidal drug program should be maximized, all underlying provoking factors should be detected and eliminated, and the corticosteroid should be reduced as soon as possible to the minimum dose that controls the asthma. Short- or intermediate-acting drugs (preferably prednisone because it is the least expensive) should be given as a single morning dose. One should attempt to switch to alternate-day therapy by giving the total dosage for 48 hours in one morning dose. If the asthma can be controlled with alternate-day steroid therapy, the side effects are usually minimal. Nevertheless, one should attempt slowly to taper even the alternate-day dose. The next best schedule is prednisone daily in the morning. In dosages of less than 15 mg/day of prednisone, side effects are generally mild and adrenal suppression is only relative (i.e., there is some response to cosyntropin).

In the unusual asthmatic who requires multiple doses of prednisone each day or a large daily dose (above 20 mg), better control may be achieved with reduced side effects by using the combination of troleandomycin and methylprednisolone. In the patient with troublesome gastrointestinal (GI) side effects, triamcinolone may be tolerated better than prednisone, but it produces more myopathy.

Drug interactions occur and should be recognized. Agents such as phenobarbital (in Tedral [Parke-Davis, Morris Plains, NJ]), phenytoin, and primidone stimulate microsomal enzymes in the liver. This increases corticosteroid metabolism, requiring a larger oral dosage of the drug but providing a much smaller effective dosage of the drug to the lung tissues.

Patient education is essential in stimulating compliance. If patients manage their own asthma by stopping and starting corticosteroids or discontinuing other supporting drugs at will, they may take more of the corticosteroid than if they had followed the original recommendation. Patients must understand the importance of avoiding provoking factors. In certain patients adverse effects of long-term corticosteroid therapy may be unavoidable. Under such circumstances the physician should inform the patient of the known adverse effects when prescribing these potent agents.

## SUGGESTED READINGS

Axelrod L: Glucocorticoid therapy. Medicine 55:39, 1976
*Nice review of effects and side effects.*
Hahn TJ, Halstead LR, Teitelbaum SL et al: Altered mineral metabolism in glucocorticoid-induced osteopenia. J Clin Invest 64:655, 1979
*Protective effects of calcium and vitamin D against osteoporosis.*
Harter RG, Reddy WJ, Thorn GM: Studies on an intermittent corticosteroid dosage regimen. New Engl J Med 269:591, 1963
*Landmark study of alternate-day prednisone treatment.*
Klinefelter HF, Winkelweder WL, Bledsoe T: Single daily dose prednisone therapy. JAMA 241:2721, 1979
*Good effects with decreased side effects from less than 15 mg of prednisone daily.*
Lockey RI: Glucocorticoids in the treatment of asthma and allergic diseases, in Lockey RF (Ed): Allergy and Clinical Immunology, Garden City, New York, Medical Exam. Publishing Co., 1979, Chapter 4, p 957
*How to use corticosteroids.*
Rimsza ME: Complications of corticosteroid therapy. Am J Dis Childh 132:806, 1978
*Side effects in children.*
Stevenson DD: Asthma, in Lockey RF (Ed): Allergy and Clinical Immunology, Garden City, New York, Medical Exam. Publishing Co., 1979, Chapter 30, p 712
*How to approach asthma and corticosteroids.*

# 11

STEPHEN I. WASSERMAN

# Use of Aerosolized Steroids in Asthma

It has been known for more than 30 years that systemic glucocorticoids are useful in the therapy of asthma, and as early as 1951 it was shown that they were also effective when administered in aerosolized form. The steroids used as aerosols (namely, cortisone acetate, prednisolone, and dexamethasone) had the same undesirable systemic effects as their oral counterparts because they were rapidly and efficiently absorbed through the mucous membranes. The development of beclomethasone dipropionate has provided a topically active agent with minimal systemic side effects because it is poorly absorbed and the small amount entering the bloodstream is rapidly metabolized by the liver into inactive products.

## PHARMACOLOGY

Beclomethasone is an alcohol-soluble white powder without taste or odor. It is administered as a microcrystalline suspension by a fluorocarbon-propelled metered-dose inhaler that delivers 42-$\mu$g of the drug in each puff.

Beclomethasone is a very potent topical agent with 5000 times the cutaneous vasoconstrictor activity of hydrocortisone. It is poorly absorbed through the skin or when given orally but it is effective when administered intravenously (IV). When more than 4 mg (equivalent to 100 puffs) is given orally, there may be a fall in the plasma cortisol indicating a systemic effect.

The plasma cortisol also is depressed after inhaled doses above 2 mg per day (about 50 puffs). In children, a fall in urinary excretion of 17-hydroxysteroids has been noted at inhaled doses of 400–800 $\mu$g/day (10–20 puffs). When given by inhalation, the drug has little effect on plasma glucose but may increase the plasma neutrophil count and depress the number of eosinophils and lymphocytes.

When it is given orally, peak absorption occurs within 6 hours, and the drug is excreted mainly in the feces with a smaller amount appearing in the urine. Approximately one-fourth of the administered dose is absorbed through the bronchial mucosa, bound to the plasma protein, and metabolized by the liver within 5 hours. Its excretion is slow, however, and detectable amounts remain in the body after 4 days.

The mechanism of action of beclomethasone dipropionate aerosol is obscure, but it is presumed to be similar to that of the systemic glucocorticoids. Among the theories proposed have been alteration in the number or ratios of adrenergic receptors, decreased metabolism of arachidonic acid, qualitative changes in leukocyte populations, and a nonspecific anti-inflammatory effect.

## CLINICAL USE

Beclomethasone dipropionate aerosol has been shown to be beneficial for patients of all ages in the treatment of asthma due to both allergic and nonallergic mechanisms. It does not seem to lose its effectiveness, even after years of continued use. It is active at doses as low as 100 µg/day (2-3 puffs) in children and 200 µg/day (5 puffs) in adults, but most studies have suggested a greater benefit for adults at doses of 400 µg/day (10 puffs). Higher doses provide even greater clinical effect but may suppress the pituitary-adrenal axis.

Improvement occurs in 70%–95% of asthmatic patients who are not steroid-dependent, and is generally noted within the first 10 days of treatment. The frequency and severity of attacks diminish, and improved pulmonary function can be demonstrated by spirometry. These effects may be potentiated by the concurrent use of other anti-asthma medications. Patients with long-standing, severe asthma appear somewhat less responsive to the drug, however. In patients not requiring systemic glucocorticoids, most experimental studies suggest that no serious pituitary-adrenal effects occur when the dose is 400–800 µg/day (8–16 puffs).

In steroid-dependent asthmatics, the use of aerosol beclomethasone dipropionate permits a decreased dose of systemic steroids and, in many cases, complete withdrawal. The effect of the aerosol is most pronounced in patients requiring the equivalent of less than 20 mg of prednisone per day, but even in those on higher doses there may be a substantial reduction in the requirement for systemic glucocorticoids. The successful transfer of a patient from systemic to aerosolized steroid is demonstrated when there is no deterioration in pulmonary function. After asthma control has been achieved with the aerosol, the dose may be decreased, but most patients continue to require 300–400 µg (8–10 puffs) per day. Flares of asthma may require temporary resumption of systemic glucocorticoid therapy. Arthralgias may be noted during withdrawal and may necessitate a prolonged, slow tapering of the systemic agent. Replacement of systemic steroids with the aerosol is associated with regression of cushingoid features and metabolic abnormalities and the return of normal pituitary-adrenal function. In addition, the aerosol does not aggravate diabetes mellitus or peptic ulcer disease.

## PROBLEMS AND SIDE EFFECTS

Inhaled beclomethasone should not be used to treat acute asthma or an exacerbation of bronchospasm. The drug is most effective when it is used as maintenance therapy after the bronchospasm is well under control. Even in asthmatics who are not steroid-dependent it may be desirable to begin treatment with a "burst" of oral prednisone for 1–2 weeks in order to clear the symptoms rapidly. Then the patient can be switched over a few days to the inhaled agent. When used as initial treatment in a patient with very irritable airways, beclomethasone often causes so much temporary cough and increased bronchospasm that it is poorly accepted even when it is preceded with an inhaled bronchodilator. In addition, with many patients it is difficult to determine whether there has been a maximal response to treatment unless the response to an adequate trial of a systemic corticoid can be evaluated. This is especially true in the adult with asthmatic bronchitis who has a major component of fixed airways obstruction in addition to bronchospasm.

It is important to instruct the patient carefully about the difference between beclomethasone and an inhaled bronchodilator. Many patients do not take their beclomethasone as frequently as prescribed because they feel that they don't need it or that it doesn't work as well as another inhaler. It must be stressed that beclomethasone is given to prevent a recurrence of bronchospasm, not to relieve acute symptoms.

The use of aerosol glucocorticoids may be associated with several problems not seen with systemic agents.

1. Malaise and arthralgias may develop during the withdrawal from oral steroids, necessitating slower reduction or even maintenance of low-dose oral glucocorticoids.
2. Allergic symptoms controlled by systemic agents (rhinitis, polyposis, atopic dermatitis) may flare up on withdrawal and require appropriate topical and systemic therapy.
3. Adrenal insufficiency and pituitary-adrenal axis abnormalities may persist, particularly in patients using aerosol and low-dose daily or alternate-day glucocorticoids.
4. Oral candidiasis is a frequent finding that usually responds quickly to topical antifungal treatment. The lesions are easily identified as red patches surrounding white plaques of fungus, most commonly located on the hard palate and faucial regions. In patients with artificial teeth it is especially common under and just behind the upper plate. The mouth should be examined with the dentures removed at every office visit. Patients should be advised to report promptly any soreness of the mouth, and such symptoms should be treated, even when there are no obvious lesions. A few days of nystatin oral suspension is usually curative. Some severe or resistant infections may respond to having the patient suck on a nystatin vaginal tablet three times daily, and it may be advisable not to wear the dentures for a few days. It is rarely necessary to discontinue the beclomethasone. Candidiasis is less of a problem if the mouth is thoroughly rinsed with water after each treatment with beclomethasone. In some patients with frequent recurrences of oral candidiasis the problem can be abolished by giving nystatin suspension 5 ml each night at bedtime.
5. Minor side effects include occasional complaints of dry mouth, hoarseness, cough, and dysphagia.

## SUGGESTED READINGS

Brown HM, Storey G, Jackson FA: Beclomethasone diproprionate aerosol in long-term treatment of perennial and seasonal asthma in children and adults: A report of five-and-half years' experience in 600 asthmatic patients. Br J Clin Pharmacol 4(suppl 3):259S–267S, 1977

Davies J, et al: Steroid-dependent asthma treated with inhaled beclomethasone diproprionate. Ann Int Med 86:549, 1977

Gaddie J, Reid IW, Skinner C: Aerosol beclomethasone dipropionate: A dose-response study in chronic asthma. Lancet 2:280, 1973

Godfrey S: The long-term evaluation of beclomethasone dipropionate in childhood asthma. Postgrad Med J 4(suppl):90, 1975

Harris DM, Martin LE, Harrison C, et al: The effect of oral and inhaled beclomethasone diproprionate on adrenal function. Clin Allergy 3:243, 1973

Milne LJR, Crompton GK: Beclomethasone dipropionate and oropharyngeal candidiasis. Br Med J 3:797, 1974

# 12

STEPHEN I. WASSERMAN

# Cromolyn Sodium in Asthma

Cromolyn sodium has been known for more than 10 years to be an effective agent for the treatment of asthma. Recent scientific advances have raised questions about its presumed mechanism of action, but as clinical experience has accumulated, the drug has gained increasing acceptance as an important addition to asthma therapy. This chapter focuses on newer aspects of cromolyn action and pharmacology as well as the spectrum of its clinical usefulness in respiratory disease.

## PHARMACOLOGY

Disodium cromoglycate was synthesized in 1965 as part of a series of studies of the biological effects of the plant extract khellin. It was shown to be effective in preventing antigen-induced bronchoconstriction in volunteer asthmatic subjects, although it has no direct bronchodilator effect. This unique property prompted commercial development of the drug.

Cromolyn is a white powder soluble in aqueous solvents at concentrations up to and exceeding 2%. Only about 1% of an oral dose is absorbed, whereas about 10% is absorbed after inhalation of the powder, and clinical reports suggest even greater absorption of aqueous aerosols of the drug. A device called a Spinhaler (Fisons Corporation, Bedford, MA) provides efficient delivery of the inhaled powder, with 50% of the dose deposited in the oropharynx and trachea, 15%–20% in the midsized bronchi, and 25%–30% in the smaller airways. The 8%–10% absorbed is sufficient to give a peak blood level of about 9 $\mu$g/ml. The drug is excreted rapidly in the urine and bile, with 75% eliminated in 2 hours and essentially 100% within 24 hours. It has a bitter taste and may provoke cough, but otherwise the drug has little or no acute toxicity in humans when given by inhalation. When it is given intravenously (IV) to dogs, doses above 5 $\mu$g/kg can produce reflex hypotension.

### Mechanism of Action

Cromolyn sodium has been extensively investigated in vivo and in vitro in a variety of animal and human model systems, each of which has provided insights into its possible modes of action, but no unifying hypothesis has emerged to explain how it exerts its beneficial effects. At the present time, evidence exists to support the hypothesis that cromolyn inhibits mast cell activation, possibly by several pathways. The mechanism by which cromolyn inhibits mediator release is unknown, but it is not due to chelation of $Ca^{2+}$ ion or to inhibition of antigen-antibody binding. Cromolyn is known to attenuate $Ca^{2+}$ ion fluxes associated with mast cell activation, to alter mast cell surface charge, to inhibit cAMP phosphodiesterase, to bind to a trypsin-sensitive site on the mast cell, and to enhance phosphorylation of a 78,000-dalton protein considered essential for inhibition of mediator release. Cromolyn is effective in preventing both the early and late phase of the allergic asthmatic response when given prior to antigen challenge.

Cromolyn is capable of abetting the transfer of water to dry air. It has been calculated that 20 mg of cromolyn could provide more than sufficient water to hydrate fully several liters of air at 37°C. Inhalation of cold or dry air is a potent bronchoconstriction stimulus in asthmatic subjects, and when the inhaled air is humidified, the bronchoconstrictive effect is blunted. Therefore, the humidifying effect of cromolyn may explain its usefulness in exercise-provoked bronchospasm. Cromolyn has also been shown to prevent broncho-constriction provoked by aerosols of sulfur dioxide and to inhibit several types of non-IgE mediated occupational asthma. These actions have led to the hypothesis that cromolyn acts directly on the "irritant" receptor. Cromolyn has also been thought to participate in various reflex arcs to cause bronchodilatation during induced bronchoconstriction. The drug, however, has no direct bronchodilator effects in either normal or asthmatic humans.

### Effects on Bronchial Hyperirritability

Finally, it has been shown that cromolyn, when used for prolonged periods, may diminish bronchoconstriction induced by aerosols of methacholine or histamine. This effect may be due to the cumulative long-term inhibition of mast cell mediator release, smooth-muscle effects, and blockade of "irritant" receptors. To date, no other drug has shown such an overall effect on bronchial irritability.

## CLINICAL USE OF CROMOLYN

Clinical experience confirms the laboratory evidence that cromolyn inhibits broncho-constriction incited by various stimuli. Cromolyn is effective in patients whose asthma is due to allergic mechanisms. It prevents asthmatic attacks in the workplace and broncho-spasm induced by cold-air inhalation, exercise, and exposure to pollutants. It is also beneficial in reducing symptoms when the cause of the attacks is unknown. Patients report decreased cough and wheeze, less need for medications (including corticosteroids), and reduced severity of attacks. They have better exercise tolerance and experience improved well-being and more restful nights. Objective evidence of benefit includes improvement in abnormal lung volumes and mechanics, and occasionally improvement in the blood gases. It is characteristic of this agent, however, that patient preference for the drug over placebo is more clear-cut than objective data might suggest. Its beneficial effects are unrelated to age, etiology of asthma, and atopic or immunotherapeutic status.

The technique of administration is important to obtain the maximum effect. Deep inspirations must be taken rather than shallow breaths in order to deliver the drug properly to the lower respiratory tract. It is a curious property of cromolyn that a favorable response may be delayed for up to 12 weeks. Therefore, it should be used for at least 2 weeks and up to 4–6 weeks if possible, before it is abandoned as ineffective. Since cromolyn may be irritating in powder form, it should not be used for patients with active asthma and is contraindicated during acute exacerbations of asthma. Stabilization of the asthma with systemic corticosteroids may be needed prior to and during the initial switch to cromolyn. Because of its low toxicity and its acceptability to many patients, its use should be considered in all asthmatics, although it is most successful in children and young adults with allergic asthma. The initial dose is 20 mg four times a day, which may be increased to a maximum of twice that amount, although few patients benefit from the higher dose. If the drug is effective, the dose may be reduced gradually to the minimum amount required to maintain the clinical response. The maintenance dose is usually 20 mg once to four times daily. In those patients whose asthmatic attacks are predictable, as occurs with exposure to animals, cold air, or exercise, 20 mg of cromolyn may be given 15–60 minutes before expected exposure.

Cromolyn solution for administration by nebulization is now available. This mode of delivery should circumvent some of the problems associated with cromolyn powder. These include the cough provoked with inhalation of the particulate cromolyn and lactose and the requirement for correct technique to use the Spinhaler (Fisons Corporation, Bedford, MA) successfully. Combination of a bronchodilator solution with the cromolyn should improve patient compliance and may also allow a trial of cromolyn for asthmatics who are not in "perfect" control. The disadvantage of this program is the additional cost and inconvenience of the apparatus needed to nebulize the solutions.

In summary, cromolyn is a valuable antiasthmatic drug that may be particularly useful in the following situations:

1. Before unavoidable exposure to known asthma triggers.
2. As a "steroid-sparing agent" in patients requiring oral or parenteral corticosteroids for asthma control.
3. In patients unresponsive to or intolerant of xanthines or beta-adrenergic agonists.
4. In patients requiring any maintenance treatment for asthma, especially if one is contemplating oral or inhaled steroids.
5. In occupational asthma.

Cromolyn is not useful and is not indicated in the treatment of acute asthma, in status asthmaticus, or in noncompliant, uncooperative patients. Naturally, it is of no benefit to patients with obstructive lung disease without a component of reversible airways obstruction.


## SIDE EFFECTS AND TOXICITY

Cromolyn is remarkably nontoxic. Sometimes it provokes cough, and patients may complain of its bitter taste. Rare reports suggest that the drug may be associated with immune-complex–like syndromes, including myositis, myalgia, arthralgia, fever, eosinophilia, and pulmonary infiltrates, or with urticaria and augmentation of bronchospasm. The mechanism of these very uncommon reactions is unknown.


## SUGGESTED READINGS

Altounyan REC: Review of clinical activity and mode of action of sodium cromoglycate. Clin Allergy 10(suppl):481–489, 1980

Church MK: Cromoglycate-like anti-allergic drugs: A review. Med Action/Drugs Today 14:281–341, 1978

Settipane GA, Klein DE, Boyd GK, et al: Adverse reactions to cromolyn. JAMA 241:811–813, 1979

Sheffer AL, Rocklin RE, Goetzl EJ: Immunologic components of hypersensitivity reactions to cromolyn sodium. New Engl J Med 293:1220–1224, 1975

Toogood JH, Lefcoe NM, Wonnacott TM, et al: Cromolyn sodium therapy—predictors of response. Adv Asthma Allergy Pulm Dis 5:2–15, 1978

## 13

DONALD D. STEVENSON

# Anticholinergic Agents

Anticholinergic drugs have been used to treat asthma for centuries. "Dr. R. Schiffmann's Asthmador powder" (R. Schiffmann Company) contains the anticholinergic drug, stramonium, which, when burned, becomes volatile and can be easily inhaled. Stramonium cigarettes have also been popular in this country. Although stramonium is seldom used in the modern treatment of asthma, several interesting observations can be made about the drug.

1. Stramonium appears to relieve asthma attacks rapidly.
2. In general, patients who respond have mild asthma and do not need other medications between their occasional asthma attacks.
3. Attacks that respond to stramonium are usually precipitated by exercise, inhalation of nonspecific irritants, or weather changes. Asthma from allergen inhalation or respiratory infections is generally not relieved by the inhalation of stramonium "smoke."
4. Smoke is irritating to any asthmatic in relapse, but smoke containing the rapid-acting anticholinergic, stramonium, counters this irritant-induced cholinergic reflex.

## CHOLINERGIC EFFECTS ON THE TRACHEOBRONCHIAL TREE

All parasympathetic efferent fibers to the tracheobronchial tree are contained in the vagus nerve, extending into central and peripheral airways and out to the terminal bronchioles. Afferent fibers originate in stretch receptors in alveoli or the irritant receptors in the tracheobronchial mucosa, traveling to the vagus nerve and then to the midbrain. Similar cough receptors in the trachea and larynx, chemoreceptors in the carotid and aortic arch, and nasosinus receptors give rise to afferent fibers that travel through different routes to the midbrain. These connections are outlined in schematic form in Figure 13-1. The reflex arc can be interrupted by either surgical excision of the vagus or by high concentrations of atropine, which blocks the cholinergic receptor.

Table 13-1 lists the effects on the tracheobronchial tree of discharge through the vagal parasympathetic fibers. Terminal bronchioles and alveolar ducts are not innervated by parasympathetic fibers and hence are not influenced by these events.

In the cholinergic dominance theory, as presented by Gold,[1,2] any stimulus, even a minimal one, activates the cholinergic afferent receptors and, as shown in Figure 13-1,

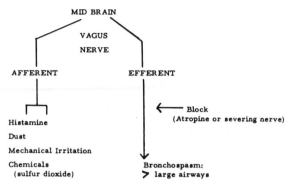

**Fig. 13-1.**   Flowchart of cholinergic action.

stimulates the cholinergic reflex arc. In asthmatics, as compared to normals, the number of receptors and their responsiveness to motor efferent impulses is exaggerated. In human asthma, this exaggerated responsiveness of the tracheobronchial tree can be demonstrated by the methacholine inhalation challenge test. Asthmatics show similar hyperreactivity when they inhale an aerosol of acetylcholine, but methacholine is used in practice because of its greater stability. Only in rare instances have inhalation challenges with methacholine (five inhalations of 50 mg/ml) failed to produce bronchospasm in patients proved to have asthma at another time. This strongly suggests that in human asthma, if minimal cholinergic stimulation of the tracheobronchial tree occurs, bronchospasm will follow. It does not prove that an increased number of impulses travel through efferent vagal fibers, resulting in the release of more acetylcholine from the postganglionic fibers in human asthmatics. Indeed, alternative explanations either of enhanced sensitivity to inhaled methacholine, or impaired beta-two adrenergic system that is incapable of countering a normal cholinergic bronchoconstrictor event are very likely. Furthermore, the cholinergic dominance theory does not exclude the operation of other pathophysiologic events, such as direct bronchial smooth-muscle response to mediators (histamines, SRS-A, prostaglandins, kinins, etc.).

## EFFECTS OF ATROPINE IN HUMANS

Atropine sulfate, scopolamine, and stramonium are available in the United States. Two synthetic quaternary ammonium compounds with more selective pharmacologic effects have been developed in England. They are atropine methylnitrate and *N*-isopropyl–nortropine–tropic acid ester methylbromide. The latter has been available in England since the 1960s, under the name of ipratropium bromide with a trade name of Atrovent (Boehringer Ingelheim Ltd., Ridgefield, CT). In the United States the same drug has been studied under investigational drug protocols, using the designation "SCH 1000," and most reports from the United States and Canada refer to it by this name.

The considerable side effects of atropine (and, by extension, all anticholinergic drugs) are summarized in Table 13-2. The side effects are dose-dependent, and overdosage causes severe, even life-threatening, toxicity. In children, ingestion of 10 mg of atropine has been fatal. Healthy adults have been known to survive doses of 1 g of atropine, despite deep coma. Atropine and its quaternary ammonium derivatives are well absorbed through mucosal surfaces. A higher concentration of the drug can be delivered to the peribronchial

Table 13-1
Effects of Parasympathetic Action on Tracheobronchial Tree

Augmentation of Mucus Gland Secretions

Stimulation of Intracellular Formation of GMP*
    Bronchial Smooth Muscle: Balance Between AMP vs GMP
        Cyclic GMP ⟶ Muscle Contraction
        Cyclic AMP ⟶ Muscle Relaxation
    Mast Cell: Balance Between GMP vs AMP
        Cyclic GMP ⟶ Augments Release of Mediators
        Cyclic AMP ⟶ Inhibits Release Mechanisms

Vasodilation in Bronchial Vascular Bed

*Cyclic guanosine 5'-monophosphate.

tissues by inhalation before excess drug spills over into the systemic circulation and begins producing side effects. Atropine sulfate cannot be given orally in a sufficient dosage to have any significant bronchial effects before systemic side effects become intolerable. Therefore, this class of drugs is the treatment of asthma administered by inhalation only.

## THERAPEUTIC EFFECTS OF ATROPINELIKE DRUGS IN HUMAN ASTHMA

The acute effects of inhaled atropinelike drugs have been studied in four types of asthma: allergic inhalant asthma, irritant inhalant asthma, exercise induced asthma, and spontaneous asthma of variable causes. In reviewing these studies, one is struck by the variety of results, ranging from complete relief of bronchospasm to no therapeutic effect. In order to understand these discrepant results, one must consider the following problems.

1. Was enough atropine (or SCH 1000) used to block cholinergic receptors adequately or completely? In general, inhaled atropine between 1 and 3 mg and Atrovent® 40–160 mg can be tolerated without significant side effects. No matter what dosage

Table 13-2
Dose-Related Side Effects of Atropine

| Dose (Oral or Parenteral) mg | Effect |
| --- | --- |
| 0.5 | Dry mouth; slowed pulse |
| 1 | Dry mouth; thirst; variable heart rate response; dilated pupils |
| 2 | Tachycardia, palpitations; very dry mouth; dilated pupils |
| 5 | Increase in above; restlessness; headache; urinary retention and decreased GI motility; dry hot skin |
| ≥10 | Delerium, coma; arrythmias |

was administered, complete cholinergic blockade has not been proved unless methacholine can be inhaled without stimulating the expected bronchospastic response.

2. Lung function measurements vary from study to study. Since the predominant effect of atropine should be on medium to large airways, those measurements, such as timed volumes ($FEV_1$) that assess the consequences of cholinergic events on large airways would be accurate and reproducible. When different studies use the $FEV_1$, however, the specific airways conductance, or the density dependent maximal flow curve (comparing flow on air and on 80% helium, 20% oxygen mixture), comparison of results is sometimes difficult.

3. Nebulization systems are not well standardized and are poorly reproducible from one study to another. Thus, efficiency of delivering drug or challenge material to the medium and large airways varies considerably.

4. Variation in design of the study and selection of patients makes it difficult to determine whether one study can be compared to another.

In the references for this section, five studies are listed[3-7] that are reasonably well done. These investigations are summarized in the following paragraphs.

*Allergic Asthma.*   Inhalation of either specific allergen or histamine can be blocked by $H_1$ antihistamine, but not by an anticholinergic (SCH 1000) drug. Most allergic asthma is produced by release of mast cell mediators that exert their effects on medium to small airways and are independent of cholinergic control.

*Irritant Inhalation.*   Bronchospasm induced by inhalation of smoke, sulfur dioxide, etc., can be blocked by pretreatment with atropine.

*Exercise.*   Pretreatment with atropine will block the bronchospasm of approximately 50% of patients with exercise-induced asthma. Deal, McFadden, Ingrahm et al.[5] have shown that in such individuals the exercise-induced asthma involves predominantly the larger airways.

A second population of asthmatics receive no protective benefit from treatment with atropine before exercise. McFadden has shown predominantly small airway obstruction in such individuals, although large airway obstruction also occurs. Simon has shown that histamine is released into the arterial circulation during exercise in one-half of exercise asthmatics patients.

Combined programs of Atrovent, cromolyn sodium, and beta-two agonists (isoproterenol, metaproterenol, fenoterol) produce the most effective and consistent protective results. These data suggest that the mechanisms of exercise induced asthma, the mediators, and their sites of action in the tracheobronchial tree vary from one patient to another. The study of small numbers of highly selected patients may produce results that cannot be applied to the entire population of asthmatics who wheeze during exercise.

*Spontaneous Asthma.*   As might be expected, some asthmatics improve after inhalation of anticholinergics, and others do not. In acute measurements over 2–4 hours, convincing evidence does not exist showing that asthma is adversely affected by drying of the bronchial mucus, causing "plugging."

In general, the use of an Atrovent inhaler (obtained from England) offers no advantage over standard beta-two inhalers (isoproterenol, metaterenol, isoetharine). However, an occasional patient receives superior and prolonged bronchodilation from inhaling Atrovent and may wish to obtain the drug from England to pretreat or treat

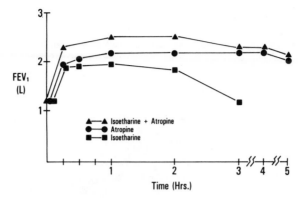

**Fig. 13-2.**   Demonstration of the effect of inhalation of atropine alone or atropine and isoetharine in combination after 5 hours of bronchodilation in selected patients. Isoetharine by itself is less effective in the patient.

irritant-induced, exercise, and spontaneous asthma attacks. Although not studied systematically, bronchospasm induced by gastroesophageal (GE) reflux also appears to benefit from anticholinergic treatment.

## LONG-TERM TREATMENT WITH ATROPINE

Adequate studies to determine whether long-term, daily inhalation of atropine is either effective or safe have not been conducted. In my practice I sometimes give patients with severe steroid-dependent asthma atropine sulfate 1 mg/ml in an aerosol nebulizer with or without a beta-2 bronchodilator and follow lung function serially for 6–8 hours. If an acute 4–6 hours potentiating bronchodilator effect can be demonstrated by improved spirometry, a home trial is indicated.

Side effects of mucosal drying and the cost of drugs are disadvantages. The response is occasionally gratifying but usually not impressive (Fig. 13-2).

## SUGGESTED READINGS

Gold WM: Cholinergic pharmacology in asthma, in Austen KF, Lichtenstein LM (Eds): Asthma: Physiology, Immunopharmacology, and Treatment. New York, Academic Press, 1973
   *Excellent presentation of the cholinergic dominance theory.*
Gold WM: Anticholinergic drugs, in Middleton, Reed C, Ellis E (Eds): Allergy: Principles and Practice. St. Louis, Mosby, 1978, Chapter 29, p 499
   *Dr. Gold presents all the facts on this subject but leans inexorably toward anticholinergics as the ultimate treatment of choice for asthmatics.*
Woenne R, Kattan M, Orange RP, et al: Bronchial hyperactivity to histamine and methocholine in asthmatic children after inhalation of SCH 1000 and chlorpheniramine. J Allergy Clin Immunol 62:119, 1978
   *Study showing histamine and methacholine are two separate stimulants for asthma. Only the latter can be blocked by SCH 1000.*

Cockcroft DW, Ruffin RE, Hargreave FE: Effect of SCH 1000 in allergen-induced asthma. Clin Allergy 8:361, 1978

   *Nice study showing that SCH 1000 does not block allergen-induced immediate hypersensitivity asthma.*

Deal EC, McFadden ER, Ingram RH, et al: Effect of atropine on potentiation of exercise-induced bronchospasm by cold air. J Appl Physiol 45:238, 1978

   *Variable effects of atropine in blocking exercise asthma.*

Thomson NC, Patel KR, Kerr JW: Sodium cromolyn glygate and ipratropium bromide in exercise-induced asthma. Thorax 33:694, 1978

   *Combination of cromolyn and Atrovent blocks all exercise-induced asthma.*

Schlueter DP, Neumann JL: Double blind comparison of acute bronchial and ventilation-perfusion changes to Atrovent and isoproterenol. Chest 73:982, 1978

   *Atrovent has a more intense and prolonged bronchodilator effect than isoproterenol.*

# 14

LAWRENCE E. KLINE

# Mucolytic Agents

Bronchospasm is often accompanied by an increased output of bronchial mucus. The narrowed bronchial lumen is more easily occluded by this mucus, and the reduced expiratory flow decreases the efficacy of cough. It would thus be desirable to have an expectorant drug for the bronchospastic patient. Unfortunately, although a number of preparations are described as "expectorant," their performance falls below the hope expressed by the name. Some of the agents that exhibit, or are alleged to exhibit, mucolytic properties are reviewed in this chapter.

An effective mucolytic agent should aid mucokinesis by diminishing the viscosity of tenacious bronchial secretions. The physcial properties of the secretions are only one factor in mucokinesis, however. They cannot be cleared from the chest unless there is adequate airflow and an effective cough.

A variety of pharmacologic agents have been used in an attempt to alter the respiratory secretions and thus improve clearance. Despite theoretical reasons for their efficacy, there is little objective evidence that they are beneficial.[1,2] Some patients do report more effective cough and easier expectoration after using these agents.

## BRONCHIAL SECRETIONS

Gelatinous mucus is discharged from goblet cells located in the bronchial epithelium. These cells have no autonomic innervation, but they are stimulated by local irritation. The tubuloacinar exocrine glands located in the bronchial submucosa of the cartilagenous bronchi are under autonomic control. These bronchial glands produce a watery fluid when stimulated by irritants, parasympathomimetics, or various drugs. The sol layer of the mucociliary blanket also contains fluid transudated from mucosal capillaries, Type II alveolar pneumocytes, and Clara cells.

Respiratory secretions tend to organize into superficial gel layer and a deeper, less vicous, sol layer. The sol layer bathes the cilia. Mucopolysaccharide is the main component of the gel layer, which traps foreign material on its sticky surface. The viscosity is determined mainly by the water content and the pH and the amount of acid glycoprotein, calcium, and cellular breakdown products such as deoxyribonucleic acid.

Mucolytic drugs affect respiratory secretions in two ways: by increasing the watery fluid content and by altering the adhesiveness or consistency of the gel layer.

103

## Hydration

Any reduction in the water content of the bronchial secretions increases their viscosity. This can be partially corrected by treating systemic dehydration with fluids and by administering inhaled aerosols of water or electrolyte solution.[3,4] Such "bland aerosols" may provoke bronchospasm in patients with reactive airways; therefore, simultaneous bronchodilator administration is advisable. Water or saline solutions can be instilled into the airways directly, or they can be nebulized. In addition to their wetting action, they stimulate bronchial glands by their irritant effect.

## Iodides

Iodides may stimulate bronchial glands directly or indirectly. The indirect action is via the gastropulmonary vagal reflex. This reflex is stimulated by subemetic amounts of emetic drugs and results in increased secretion by the bronchial glands. Other suggested actions of iodides are a direct mucolytic action on glycoproteins, potentiation of proteases in secretions, and excitation of the cilia.

The usefulness of iodide therapy is limited by a variety of adverse effects that include gastric irritation, cutaneous reactions, hypersensitivity, angioedema, thyroid dysfunction, and iodism (acneform rash, parotitis, fever, and rhinitis). Although reported side effects are numerous, serious toxicity is rare.

Iodides are available in inorganic and organic preparations.[5] It may take a week or more of therapy with either to achieve the maximum effect.

The two major inorganic preparations are sodium iodide and potassium iodide. The former can be given intravenously (IV) in a dose of 1–3 g over 24 hours. Potassium iodide is usually given as a saturated solution (SSKI) that contains 1 g of iodide per milliliter of solution and 6 meq of potassium. The recommended daily dose of SSKI is 25–35 mg/kg, but it is frequently given in doses of up to 10 drops (1 ml or 1 g) four times a day. Potassium iodide is also available in 300-mg tablets.

If the inorganic preparations are not well tolerated, an organic iodide can be tried. It is claimed that iodinated glycerol (e.g., Organidin [Wallace Laboratories, Cranbury, NJ]) is better tolerated and effective in a lower total dose. For adults, a dose of 30–60 mg four times a day can be used and for children, half the adult dose.

A few days of treatment with iodide preparations may be justifiable in a patient who is having difficulty raising tenacious secretions. Long-term treatment is rarely advisable because of the high incidence of thyroid dysfunction and other side effects, and the marginal benefits, if any, of such therapy.

## Guaifenesin

Guaifenesin (glyceryl guaiacolate) enjoys popularity in excess of any evidence of its effectiveness. If it has any influence on bronchial secretion, it probably acts in subemetic doses by stimulating the gastropulmonary vagal reflex described previously. Side effects are few except for nausea and vomiting. Diminished platelet aggregation and false positive urine test for 5-hydroxyindolacetic acid have been reported. The usual dose in adults is 100–200 mg every 3–4 hours, although up to 2400 mg/day has been recommended by some physicians.

## Sodium Bicarbonate

Sodium bicarbonate[5] may also improve the viscosity of respiratory tract secretions. Alkaline solutions tend to make mucus less adhesive and to activate natural proteases present in purulent sputum. Hypertonic solutions can also increase the volume of respiratory secretion by their osmotic effect and by irritation. The activity of acetylcysteine may be enhanced, but many bronchodilators are inactivated in an alkaline environment. Concentrations greater than 2% tend to be more irritating. Doses of 1–3 ml of a 2% solution can be used every 4–8 hours by direct instillation, or as an aerosol. If tolerated, 5% and 7.5% solutions can be used in the same way.

## Acetylcysteine (Mucomyst)

Acetylcysteine and the proteolytic enzymes[4] do have a true mucolytic action in vitro. The former is much more widely used. It contains free sulfhydryl groups that interact with the disulfide bridges of mucoprotein, causing it to be less viscous. The hydrogen sulfide product of this reducing agent explains the characteristic odor. It has more action on mucoid than on purulent secretions. In many patients, especially asthmatics, it provokes cough or bronchospasm. A marked bronchorrhea may also occur, which can be a problem if it is not expectorated adequately. Acetylcysteine is also more effective when in an alkaline (pH 7–9) environment and thus is less active in the low pH of most bronchodilator solutions and in the acidic conditions of the lung.

Acetylcysteine can be administered orally or intravenously, or by inhalation or direct instillation.[6] The last two methods are the most commonly used. When nebulized, a dose of 3–5 ml of the 20% or 6–10 of the 10% solution can be used three to four times a day.

## Deoxyribonuclease (Dornase)

Deoxyribonuclease is a mucolytic enzyme specific for deoxyribonucleic acid. It has little effect on mucoprotein or fibrin. This agent is thought to be most useful in viscid, purulent secretions. Although proteolytic agents such as trypsin can damage living tissue, Dornase does not. Nevertheless, tissue irritation, bronchospasm, and hypersensitivity reactions do occur. It should not be used in patients allergic to beef protein.

The recommended dose is 50,000–100,000 units in 2 ml of normal saline four times a day for 2–3 days.

## FINAL NOTE

A long list of agents has been used in the past for their supposed mucokinetic effect. Many have been removed from the market, some are used with little if any proof of efficacy, and others have an unfavorable risk–benefit balance. The agents discussed represent those that might be beneficial in selected patients. Clearly, more systematic study of mucolytic agents is necessary to help define their proper place in the management of asthma.

# REFERENCES

1. Wanner A, Aswath R: Clinical indications for and effect of bland, mucolytic and antimicrobial aerosals. Am Rev Respir Dis 122:79, 1980
2. Wanner A: Clinical aspects of mucociliary transport. State of the Art. Am Rev Respir Dis 116:73, 1977
3. Richard J: Effect of relative humidities in the rheologic properties of bronchial mucus. Am Rev Respir Dis 109:484, 1974
4. Yeager H: Tracheobronchial secretions. Am J Med 50:493, 1971
5. Ziment I: Mucokinetic agents, in Zigment I (Ed): Respiration Pharmacology and therapeutics, Philadelphia, Saunders, 1978, Chapter 3.
6. Donaldson J, Stoop D, Raymond L, et al: Acetylcystein for life-threatening acute bronchial obstruction. Ann Int Med 88:656, 1978

# 15

Donald D. Stevenson

# Avoidance and Immunotherapy

Atopy is the immunologic mechanism responsible for hay fever and allergic asthma. These are also called immune (IgE-antibody-recognized) hypersensitivity reactions, as contrasted to nonimmunologic hypersensitivity reactions that occur when certain drugs (codeine) or radiographic contrast media directly combine with mast cell membranes to release histamine and other mediators.

In 1963, Gell and Coombs[1] proposed a classification for immune-mediated reactions. These are listed in Table 15-1.

Figure 15-1 shows the components of an immune-recognized immediate hypersensitivity reaction (Type I, Gell and Coombs).

It should be observed that the antigen (allergenic particle) may be inhaled (pollen grains, dust particles, animal danders, mold spores, insect emanations, flour, etc.), ingested (food, drug, mold, etc.), or injected (insect venom, drug). When antigen combines with antibody fixed to mast cells or basophiles, histamine and other mediators are released into the surrounding tissues or fluids. The concentration of these mediators will thus be greatest at their sites of release. Another variable is shock organ sensitivity or responsiveness to chemical mediators and is the important variable in determining which shock organs will respond to mediator assault. For allergic asthma to occur, the following sequence must be activated:

1. Genetic propensity toward atopy.
2. Exposure to extrinsic allergens (e.g., cat dander).
3. Immunocytes synthesizing specific IgE antibody that recognizes (cat antigen). Allergy skin tests to cat extract become positive.
4. Unknown assault (? viral infection) produces responsive bronchial tree (asthma).
5. Patient exposed to cat inhalants, IgE recognizes, mast cells release mediators which activate an asthmatic attack.

## PREVALENCE OF ALLERGIC (IgE) ASTHMA

One of the most comprehensive epidemiologic studies in the United States for probable and suspected asthma was carried out in Tecumseh, Michigan. Broder et al.[2] discovered a total potential population of 12.5% asthmatics in the 11,305-member study community. Transposed into the total population of the United States, there should be about 25 million asthmatics in the country. Many of these individuals have mild allergic or exercise asthma that they treat with over-the-counter medications. It is estimated that only

**Table 15-1**
**Immune-Mediated Reactions**

| Type | Reaction |
|------|----------|
| I | IgE (reagin) anaphylactic |
| II | Cytotoxic; IgG plus complement and cell membrane antigen |
| III | Immune complex disease |
| IV | Delayed or lymphocyte-mediated disease |

9 million asthmatics are treated in the U.S. medical care delivery system. At Scripps Clinic, we have had an opportunity to consecutively study 234 adult and childhood asthmatics presenting to our allergy division.[3] Of these, 45% had IgE-mediated asthma. However, in only 25% of the 234 patients was IgE-mediated asthma the major mechanism in the pathogenesis of that patient's asthma. Only 5% of the patients had pure IgE-mediated asthma with no other provoking factor. It is this 5–25% subset of asthmatics with important IgE-mediated asthma who can be treated with either avoidance of specific allergens[4] or immunotherapy with specific allergens.

## AVOIDANCE

Cutaneous tests with extracts of environmental allergens produce wheal-and-flare responses to those allergens against which specific IgE antibodies are directed. When possible, avoidance of those allergens producing positive wheal-and-flare responses is appropriate. The converse is also true, since avoidance of allergens to which one is not

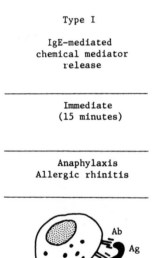

Type I

IgE-mediated
chemical mediator
release

Immediate
(15 minutes)

Anaphylaxis
Allergic rhinitis

Ab

Ag

mediators

**Fig. 15-1.**  Type I immune-recognized immediate hypersensitivity reaction.

allergic is both useless and inappropriate. Complete avoidance of a specific allergen eliminates IgE reactions for that allergen. Partial avoidance reduces the consequences of antigen–IgE interaction. Cumulative effects are also important. Avoidance is generally most successful within houses. From within the home, the inhaled substances most likely to provoke IgE-triggered asthma include house dust mite, animal proteins, and fungal spores.[4]

## House Dust

House dust usually contains fibrous materials of plant and synthetic origin; human epidermis; fungi; bacteria; food remnants; inorganic substances; mites; and in some households, proteins from domestic pets and cockroach or other insect parts. Within the past decade, mites of the genus *Dermatophagoides* have been shown to be a major allergen in house dust. This allergen is concentrated in fecal particles that are 10–40 m in diameter. Bed and bedroom floor dust ordinarily contain the highest concentrations of mite allergen. Antidust programs are designed to remove or cover dust-generating materials. Since optimal growth of *Dermatophagoides* occurs at 25°C and 75%–80% relative humidity, live mite populations tend to be greatest during warm and humid months and in homes where relative humidity is over 45%. The populations vary inversely with altitude with none found at altitudes greater than 1600 m. Concentrations of airborne mite allergen increase with activity in the home and probably increase with operation of forced-air heating systems.

## Animal Danders

Specific avoidance of outdoor animals (horses, cows, sheep) or birds (chickens, turkeys, pigeons) may be necessary in specifically sensitive individuals.

Household pets, including cats, dogs, and rodents, disseminate aeroallergens in the form of proteins desquamated from their skin epithelium or excreted in saliva or urine. Individual hypersensitivity to these proteins may be exquisite in that even brief exposures in households occupied by animals may precipitate severe asthma. Avian proteins encountered from feather pillows or down comforters may also trigger asthmatic attacks in hypersensitive individuals. Eviction of pets and replacement of pillows is appropriate.

## Fungal Spores

Airborne spores are generated from fungi that grow in predominantly microscopic cultures in moist areas of the home, including food storage areas, garbage containers, soiled upholstery, carpets, rubber and synthetic foams, and soil and drainage pans of overwatered house plants. Poorly maintained cold-mist vaporizers and console humidifiers may emit dense fungus aerosols. Damage from breaks in waterlines or floods to carpets and floors produces an environment highly conducive to proliferation of fungi. Small-spored (2–3-$\mu$m) species of *Penicillium* and *Aspergillus, Rizopus,* and *Mucor* as well as unicellular yeasts ordinarily dominate the microflora within the household; however, outdoor spore clouds (*Alternaria, Cladosporum,* and *Helminthosporium* are the most numerous of the genera known to be allergenic) also readily penetrate the household except during snowcover. Antimold programs are designed to destroy mold and thus reduce spores. These results are achieved by denying molds either substrate or moisture and/or by killing molds with fungicidal chemicals.

Other aeroallergens occasionally encountered in the household that may be relevant to an individual's asthma include allergens of plant origin such as the seed hair of kapok trees employed as stuffing for pillows or mattresses, cottonseed contaminants of inexpensive cotton stuffing in upholstery and cushions, lycopodium dusting powders, psyllium laxatives, and jute carpets. Fish and other airborne food molecules generated during cooking can produce asthmatic symptoms in highly sensitive patients. For spore- and/or pollen-sensitive patients, window or central air conditioners will substantially reduce indoor allergen levels (and presumably disease) by maintaining relative isolation from outdoor spores and pollens and to lesser extents by reducing relative humidity and air filtration. To be maximally effective, outside air should be excluded from the system and filters cleaned or replaced regularly. Addition of a high-efficiency central air cleaner may add minimal improvement.

Air exchanged through central air filters only approximates the air that enters the home from the outdoors; thus only a 50% improvement in air purity is achieved. A high-volume high-efficiency particulate air (HEPA) cleaner room unit offers the potential for reducing particulates in the room by 90%.


## IMMUNOTHERAPY

Repeated subcutaneous injections of increasing concentrations of allergy extracts to which the patient has allergic (IgE) antibody gradually desensitizes (i.e., renders that individual less sensitive) to the reintroduction of the antigens through natural routes of entry. The specific technique is well described by Patterson et al.[5] There are three issues that seem important in a decision to use immunotherapy: (1) whether immunotherapy is effective in decreasing sensitivity in patients with hay fever and asthma, (2) whether immunotherapy is safe, and (3) whether the results are worth the cost, time, and long-term commitment.


### Efficacy of Immunotherapy

Since 1949, there have been over 20 double-blind–placebo controlled immunotherapy studies for efficacy. Of the placebo-treated groups, 20%–30% improved, and 60%–80% of the allergen treated groups were shown to improve when the combined results were summarized. Two studies have shown no effect from immunotherapy, but their design, patient selection, dose of extracts used, and analysis of data differ and to some critics represent the prestudy bias of the investigators. Most studies have analyzed the effects of immunotherapy on hay fever or insect venom sensitivity. Only two studies have analyzed the effect of immunotherapy on the course of asthma (see Table 15-2).

Both studies show that immunotherapy is effective in groups of children who had allergic asthma and a low probability of simultaneously experiencing other types of asthma, except intercurrent respiratory infections and exercise-induced asthma. Similar studies have not been conducted in adults. However, there is no evidence that IgE-mediated asthma in adults is different from that found in children. On the basis of the studies for hay fever, limited studies in asthmatics and clinical assessment, aqueous immunotherapy is effective in decreasing sensitivity to inhaled allergens in allergic asthmatics.

Table 15-2
Immunotherapy Treatment for Asthma

| Study | Years | Placebo Therapy | | Allergen Therapy | |
|---|---|---|---|---|---|
| | | +/N | % | +/N | % |
| Johnstone and Dutton (6) | 10–14 | 16/63 | 25 | 51/67 | 76 |
| Tuchinda and Chai* (7) | 1 | 0/5 | 0 | 10/10 | 100 |

*Improvement measured by repeat bronchial inhalation challenges.

## Safety of Immunotherapy

Over 70 years of experience with aqueous immunotherapy has shown no long-term adverse effects from this treatment. Specific surveys for appearance of cancer or immunodeficiency diseases have failed to demonstrate such problems in treated populations. One controversial study from the University of Colorado reports a relationship between initiating immunotherapy and the onset of polyarteritis nodosum. The major criticisms of this report involve the small numbers of patients, the failure to prove that polyarteritis was absent before immunotherapy was activated, and the self-selection of polyarteritis through referral patterns and author interest. Reasonably astute clinicians at other institutions have been unable to identify polyarteritis in populations of patients receiving long-term immunotherapy. Surveys for production of nuclear antibody (ANA) in treated populations have failed to demonstrate an increased incidence of these antibodies.

Short-term side effects from immunotherapy are local and systemic reactions to the injected allergens. Local reactions at the injection site occur in most patients receiving immunotherapy as top treatment dosage is approached. Adequacy of dosage is based in part on observation of this phenomenon. Systemic anaphylaxis is not desired but when it does occur, it is usually mild, and responds quickly to a subcutaneous injection of aqueous adrenalin. The circumstances where systemic anaphylaxis are most likely to occur are (1) as a result of overdosage (wrong dosage), (2) during buildup or increasing injections, and (3) when the patient has an increased circulation (exercise or fever). In most allergy clinics one in 500 injections produces a systemic reaction, depending on what criteria are used to define systemic reaction.

## CRITERIA FOR SELECTING ASTHMATIC PATIENTS FOR IMMUNOTHERAPY

Of the 234 asthmatic patients in our Scripps Clinic study, approximately 50% had positive wheal-and-flare skin tests. Therefore, the 50% with negative wheal-and-flare skin tests did not have any allergies and were automatically not candidates for immunotherapy. Of the 50% with positive skin tests, only one-half of these (25%) of the total group of 234 asthma patients have major or important allergic components operative in the pathogenesis of their asthma. Of this smaller group, less than one-half (10%) of the 234 are candidates for immunotherapy.

This 10% group of asthmatics has significant allergic asthma and are unable to avoid their allergens or block their effects with simple medication programs that do not in themselves produce side effects. Those factors on which our recommendation of immuno-

**Table 15-3**
**Potential Immunotherapy Programs**

---

Modified allergens to reduce reactions and number of injections
    Alum precipitation
    Glutaraldehyde-polymerized allergens
    Formalin-modified (allergoids)

Mucosal immunization combined with aldehyde-polymerized allergens (nasal inhalation daily)

Tolerogens—induction of IgE tolerance
    Urea-denatured antigens: T-cell suppression
    Polyethylene glycol-substituted allergens: T-cell suppression
    Synthetic Copolymer of 2-D-glutamic and D-lysine amino acids (D-GL) arranged in
    random linear sequence—conjugated with antigens: producing B-cell tolerance

---

therapy is based are as following:

1. Significant asthma.
2. Associated hay fever, particularly with complications (sinusitis, postnasal drainage, cough).
3. Allergens that cannot be avoided.
4. Side effects from medications used to treat asthma/hay fever.
5. Childhood allergic asthma.
6. Favorable response to immunotherapy in other family members.
7. Skin tests are positive at high dilution of antigen extracts.

    Most immunotherapy programs are continued for a minimum of 5 years with weekly injections the first year, 2-week intervals the second year, 3-week intervals the third year, and 4-week intervals for fourth and fifth years. Motivation for each patient to complete or discontinue the program will likely be related to (1) Degree of improvement, (2) ease of receiving the injections, (3) financial coverage, (4) acceptance or dislike of alternative treatment options—medications, etc., and (5) geographic stability.

## Future of Immunotherapy

    There are a number of promising chemical modifications of extract antigens which have potential in either improving immune response of blocking antibody, decreasing local and systemic reactions, and/or arresting synthesis of specific IgE antibodies. Studies using these modified extracts are under way. Table 15-3 lists some new approaches.

    Until these improved extracts have completed trials for efficacy and safety, continued use of aqueous antigen extracts is appropriate. In contrast, so called bacterial vaccines have been shown in definitive trials not to have any therapeutic benefit in the course of treating asthmatics.

## REFERENCES

1. Gell PGH and Coombs RRA: The classification of allergic reactions underlying disease, in Gell PGH and Coombs RRA (Eds) *Clinical Aspects of Immunology.* Philadelphia, FA Davis, 1964, Chapter 13, p 317.

2.   Broder I, Higgins MW, Mathews KP, et al: Epidemiology of asthma and allergic rhinitis in a total community, Tecumseh, Michigan. J Allergy Clin Immunol 53:127, 1974

*In a farming community of 11,305 the authors discovered a cumulative prevalence for asthma of 6.5% (probable) and 6.0% (suspected) for a total potential prevalence of 12.5%.*

3.   Stevenson DD, Mathison DA, Tan, EM et al: Provoking factors in bronchial asthma. Arch Int Medi 35:777, 1975

*A study of 234 consecutive asthmatic patients at Scripps Clinic. Patients were divided into subsets on the basis of provoking factors and mechanisms.*

4.   Mathison DA, Stevenson DD, Simon RA: Asthma and the home environment. Editorial, Ann Int Med 97:128, 1982

*A review of avoidance therapy for the treatment of IgE-mediated respiratory disease.*

5.   Patterson R, Lieberman P, Irons JS et al: Immunotherapy, in Middleton EL, Reed CR, Ellis EF (Eds): Allergy: Principles and Practice, St. Louis, Mosby, 1978, Chapter 49, p 877

*Thorough review of subject (history, efficacy, mechanisms of effect, practice, future treatments).*

6.   Johnstone DE, Dutton A: The value of hyposensitization therapy for bronchial asthma in children—a 14 year study. Pediatrics 42:793, 1968

*Only double blind study of immunotherapy and its effect on asthma; 25% of placebo treated and 76% of antigen treated asthmatics went into remission of asthma during the 10–14 years of treatment.*

7.   Tuchinda Mi, Chai, H. Effect of immunotherapy in chronic asthmatic children. J Allergy Clin Immunol 51:131, 1973

*Allergen inhalation challenge before and after 12 months of immunotherapy or placebo showed that 10 of 10 (100%) allergen-treated patients were protected from adverse effects of the second allergen challenge after therapy.*

## SUGGESTED READINGS

Katz DH: Control of IgE antibody production by suppressor substances. J Allergy Clin Immunol 62:44, 1978

*Review of future approach to controlling IgE antibody synthesis with new modified vaccines.*

Zeiss CR: Immunotherapy in allergic disease, in Lockey RF (Ed): Allergy and Clinical Immunology, Garden City, New York, Medical Exam. Publishing Co., 1979, Chapter 42, p 977

*Beautiful review of the subject.*

# 16

LAWRENCE E. KLINE

# Antimicrobial Agents: Management of Acute Infection in the Asthmatic

Antimicrobial agents play a minor role in the therapy of asthma. Although infections of the upper or lower respiratory tract are frequently associated with exacerbations of asthma, they are usually of viral rather than bacterial origin.[1-3]

Antibiotics should be given if pathogenic bacteria are identified in purulent secretions, but their routine use in asthmatics is unjustified. Specific agents and their application are discussed later.

## PREVENTIVE MEASURES

Vaccines to prevent infection are useful in the asthmatic. The pneumococcal vaccine contains antigens of 14 common strains and is an effective prophylaxis in most patients. It reduces the incidence of pneumonia, otitis media, and meningitis caused by this organism. The pneumococcal vaccine is safe and effective, but local and systemic reactions are more likely to occur in healthy adults if they are given a second dose. The time requirement for revaccination and the optimal dose for revaccinating have not yet been established. The pneumococcal vaccine has been recommended for patients with a number of chronic diseases, including asthma and for selected healthy persons over 50 years old.[4,5] It is not advised during pregnancy or in children under 2 years old.

The risk of exacerbations of asthma caused by the influenza virus can be reduced with the flu vaccine and with amantidine[6-8] therapy. The flu vaccine should be given annually, especially in the chronic or severe asthmatic, even though it can occasionally produce an exacerbation. It should not be given during an acute febrile illness. Adverse reactions from the flu vaccine have received much publicity, but serious problems are rare.

Minor reactions to the influenza vaccine include fever, malaise and myalgia, and a flulike syndrome. This begins 6–12 hours after the immunization and lasts for 1–2 days. It is self-limiting and is rarely a serious problem. A second problem is a hypersensitivity reaction generally related to egg protein.

A very rare but major complication of influenza vaccination is the Guillain-Barre syndrome. This is an ascending paralysis, which is usually self-limiting. During the 1976 mass vaccination against swine flu, there were 10 cases per million vaccinations, which added up to a five- to sixfold greater risk of this disease than that seen in the unvaccinated population. Since 1978 the incidence of Guillain-Barre syndrome was no different in unvaccinated and vaccinated individuals.

Amantidine was originally released for the treatment of Parkinson's disease, but it is an antiviral agent effective only against influenza A2. The daily dose is 200 mg in one or two doses. The divided dose may reduce the central nervous system (CNS) side effects such as confusion, dizziness, slurred speech, and sleep disturbance that are occasionally seen in the elderly or in patients with renal insufficiency. Fluid retention can occur with chronic use. Adverse reactions generally occur within 48 hours and usually disappear promptly when the drug is discontinued.

There are three situations where amantidine should be considered. The first is for prophylaxis during known epidemics. Previous flu vaccination may enhance the effectiveness of the drug. Since community outbreaks tend to extend over intervals of 4–12 weeks, this is an adequate duration of therapy. If it is continued throughout the period of exposure, it can prevent clinical infection in 70%–100% of adults. The flu vaccine can be administered simultaneously with amantidine to those patients who have not received it. In 2–3 weeks the antibody response will be adequate and the amantidine can be discontinued unless its added benefit is desired for high-risk patients.

The second type of usage is for a patient with known exposure to influenza A. Here amantidine should be continued for 10 days after exposure to the virus. The third situation is for the patient who has symptoms of flu. Amantidine should be started as early as possible and can be used for 1–2 days after symptoms disappear.

## ANTIBACTERIAL THERAPY DURING AN EXACERBATION OF ASTHMA

In the patient with uncomplicated asthma, acute respiratory infections should be treated with antibacterial agents according to the same principles that would apply in the otherwise healthy population. Fever, leukocytosis with a left shift, and purulent secretions may suggest bacterial infection, but these are not diagnostic findings. The Gram stain can be very useful in suggesting a bacterial pathogen, but sputum and nasal secretions are often contaminated with nasal and pharyngeal flora. For this reason, some have questioned the value of routine sputum cultures,[9] but in selected patients they are helpful since bacterial infections are so infrequent in asthmatics. When the sputum is very purulent and a dominant pathogen is suggested by the Gram stain, it may be desirable to start antibacterial treatment without awaiting the culture report. Occasionally the Gram stain and culture can specifically identify a pathogen, sometimes an unusual one.

Radiologic studies of the paranasal sinuses and the chest should be considered when the clinical findings suggest suppurative sinusitis or pneumonia.

Antibiotic therapy is appropriate when there is evidence of an infection amenable to treatment. *Streptococcus pneumoniae* and *Haemophilus influenzae* are two frequent bacterial pathogens, but both may be part of normal oropharyngeal flora. Other bacterial pathogens, *Mycoplasma pneumoniae,* and certain fungi may also require treatment. Antibacterial agents should not be used routinely to treat an exacerbation of asthma when there are no findings to indicate bacterial infection.

## ANTIBACTERIALS IN CHRONIC BRONCHITIS

The approach to chronic bronchitis and emphysema is somewhat different. Antibiotic therapy is not based on clear bacteriologic principles. The role of bacterial infection, the selection of an antibiotic, and the duration of therapy are the subject of controversy.[10-12] In some studies short courses of antibiotics have resulted in clinical improvement, prevention of deterioration, clearing of sputum purulence, and eradication of organisms when compared with placebo.[13] Sputum pathogens have not been consistently identified in exacerbations of chronic bronchitis.[14] Although antibiotic treatment appears valuable in some clinical studies, the microbiologic basis for this is unclear and routine sputum cultures are not generally needed.[15] Tetracycline, ampicillin, and trimethoprin-sulfa-methoxazole are the agents most commonly used for such empiric therapy, but a recent controlled study of tetracycline therapy for exacerbations of chronic bronchitis suggested no advantage over placebo.[16] Perhaps the methods used to evaluate the microbial ecology of the respiratory tract and variations between studies of how an exacerbation of chronic bronchitis was defined contribute to the controversy. Nevertheless, antibiotic therapy seems reasonable for life-threatening exacerbations of chronic bronchitis.[17]

Most chest specialists are willing to treat the patient with an exacerbation of chronic obstructive lung disease with an antibiotic without bacteriological studies. The asthmatic generally should not be given antibiotic treatment unless there is supportive evidence of a bacterial infection. Future studies may resolve this seeming paradox. One could speculate that in chronic obstructive lung disease there is colonization of the respiratory tract by organisms that are not ordinarily considered pathogenic but that contribute to the inflammatory process. Perhaps the clearance of secretions and the resolution of symptoms can be hastened if these organisms are eradicated with a broad-spectrum antibiotic. The clinical studies done thus far may not have been adequate in identifying a slight beneficial effect of antibacterial treatment. These and other questions are yet to be clearly answered.

Patients with chronic suppurative sinusitis can benefit from antibacterial agents, but they may also require surgical treatment such as maxillary antral windows, Caldwell-Luc, or other drainage procedures.

## ANTIBIOTIC SELECTION

The selection of an antibiotic is based on a number of considerations. The first is the organism identified and its drug sensitivity. The clinical situation, the Gram stain, and appropriate radiographs usually provide enough information on which to base an early choice. Definite identification of a pathogen and determination of its drug sensitivity takes from a few days to a few weeks, depending on the organism. This may confirm the original choice of antibiotic or dictate a change of drugs, but therapy should not be delayed until the culture report is available if there is strong clinical evidence of a bacterial infection. Naturally, the reliability of the information depends on the quality of the specimen and of the laboratory.

A review of therapy for unusual infections such as fungi, mycobacteria, or rare bacterial pathogens is beyond the scope of this chapter. In addition, the parenteral treatment of severe infections or of debilitated patients is not reviewed. The majority of asthmatics are ambulatory, and the oral agents used in the adult outpatient setting are discussed.

### Ampicillin, Amoxicillin, and Bacampicillin

*H. influenzae* and *S. pneumoniae* are the two common bacterial pathogens that may exacerbate an asthmatic attack. Ampicillin is the drug of choice for the former and effective also against the latter. Amoxicillin and bacampicillin are better absorbed from the gastrointestinal (GI) tract and, in our experience, better tolerated than ampicillin. Blood levels for amoxicillin are over twice those achieved with ampicillin. Blood levels for amoxicillin can achieve even higher serum concentrations with a comparable dose. Since drug concentrations in respiratory secretions are related to serum concentration, this can be an advantage.[18] Bacampicillin tends to concentrate in bronchial secretions better than ampicillin or amoxicillin.[19,20] Ampicillin is less expensive than amoxicillin, but the cost difference is not excessive. A regimen of 2 g/day of ampicillin for 2 weeks costs approximately $10.85, compared to $14.80 for amoxicillin for the same duration at 750 mg/day. Bacampicillin in a dose of 400 mg twice a day for 2 weeks costs $32.30. The convenience of a twice-daily dose and higher concentration in bronchial secretions offers a potential advantage that must be balanced against the substantially increased cost.

### The Tetracyclines

When *H. influenzae* infections are resistant to amoxicillin, trimethoprim-sulfamethoxazole or tetracycline should be used rather than chloramphenicol.[21] Tetracycline is effective against the pneumococcus, although resistant strains are frequently seen. Tetracycline is also useful for *M. pneumoniae* infections. The long-acting and short-acting tetracyclines do not differ in their antimicrobial effectiveness. Oxytetracycline is shorter-acting and is associated with less diarrhea. The longer-acting tetracyclines such as doxycycline (Vibramycin [Pfizer Inc., New York, NY]) can be given in one or two doses and concentrate well in respiratory secretions.[22] The cost difference between tetracyclines is significant (see Table 16-1). A 2-week course of tetracycline costs $5.80, compared to $32.50 for doxycycline. Gastrointestinal (GI) intolerance with nausea and diarrhea are the most frequent side effects. The tetracyclines are better absorbed if they are taken on an empty stomach. These agents should not be used during pregnancy or in children under the age of 8 because of the risk of interference with normal development of the teeth.

The dose of tetracycline is 500 mg, three to four times a day in adults. Doxycycline is used in a dose of 100 mg once or twice a day.

### Trimethoprim-Sulfamethoxazole

An excellent alternative for both *H. influenzae* and *S. pneumoniae* infections is trimethoprim-sulfamethoxazole (TMP-SMZ). This antibacterial combination was initially introduced for the treatment of urinary infections, but it has also proven effective in

**Table 16-1**
**Antimicrobial Agents**

| Antibiotic | 2-Week Course | Cost |
| --- | --- | --- |
| Ampicillin | 500 mg qid | $10.85 |
| Amoxicillin | 500 mg tid | $14.80 |
| Bacampicillin | 400 mg q12h | $32.30 |
| Tetracycline | 500 mg qid | $ 5.80 |
| Doxycycline | 100 mg q12h | $35.20 |
| TMP-SMZ DS* | 1 Tablet q12h | $17.45 |
| Erythromycin | 500 mg qid | $13.85 |
| Cephalexin | 500 mg qid | $56.00 |
| Cefaclor | 500 mg qid | $82.50 |

*DS = double strength.
TMP-SMZ = Trimethoprim-Sulfamethoxazole

treating infections of the upper and lower respiratory tracts. In one study it was superior to ampicillin in reducing sputum purulence and volume.[23]

A variety of adverse reactions can limit the usefulness of TMP-SMZ. They include nausea, vomiting, skin eruptions, hypersensitivity reactions, and, rarely, hematologic and CNS toxicity. Due to the reports of teratogenicity, sulfa drugs should be avoided in pregnant women.

Each tablet of TMP-SMZ contains 80 mg of trimethoprim and 400 mg of sulfamethoxazole. Two regular-strength or one double-strength tablet every 12 hours is the recommended dose. Higher doses have been recommended for exacerbations of chronic bronchitis without much supporting evidence.[24]

## Erythromycin

Erythromycin is less effective for *H. influenzae* than the previously mentioned drugs, but it is effective against *S. pneumoniae* and *M. pneumoniae*. The estolate form is the only derivative well absorbed orally and can be given with food. It can cause a variety of adverse effects, including abdominal cramps, nausea, vomiting, and diarrhea. Cholestatic jaundice is uncommon and resolves rapidly with cessation of treatment. The adult dose of erythromycin estolate ranges from 250 to 500 mg four times a day.

Erythromycin and troleandomycin are both macrolide antibiotics. Troleandomycin potentiates the effect of glucocorticoids and increases the half-life of theophylline. There have been conflicting reports in the recent literature on whether erythromycin delays the metabolism of theophylline. Until this question is resolved, it is probably a wise precaution to lower the dose of theophylline by 30% if erythromycin is started in a patient receiving a therapeutic dose of theophylline.

## Cephalosporins

There are currently three oral forms of cephalosporin antibiotics in general use—cephalexin, cephradine, and cefaclor.[25] Cephalexin and cephradine are not reliable for treating *H. influenzae,* but cefaclor is active against this organism. Adverse effects with the cephalosporins include fever, rash, and hypersensitivity reactions, but there is less GI intolerance than with the other drugs mentioned. The suggested dose of these agents is approximately 2 g/day in divided doses.

## COST CONSIDERATIONS

Comparing the cost of antibiotics is difficult because the prices charged by pharmacies vary a good deal. Table 16-1 lists approximate prices from a representative San Diego pharmacy. The cost of a 2-week course of cephalexin given at 2 g/day is $56.00. Cefaclor is $82.50, $26.00 more than cephalexin at the same dose. At the suggested doses given for each agent, note the comparison for 2 weeks of treatment. Ampicillin is $10.50, amoxicillin is $14.80, bacampicillin is $32.30, tetracycline is $5.80, doxycycline is $35.20, trimethoprim-suflamethoxazole DS is $17.40, and erythromycin is $13.85.

## SUMMARY

Acute viral upper or lower respiratory infections frequently accompany exacerbations of asthma. Bacterial infections are much less common; thus antibiotic therapy should not be used routinely. *H. influenzae* and *S. pneumoniae* are the most likely bacterial pathogens. A Gram stain and culture of purulent secretions are appropriate before initiating antibiotics, unless the patient has chronic obstructive lung disease. With COPD, a broad-spectrum antibiotic is more frequently necessary and the laboratory studies are less useful.[26] Since antibiotics are seldom necessary in the asthmatic, microbiology studies should be done to help determine the need for this form of therapy. Antibiotic therapy is no substitute for measures to control the bronchospasm including short term corticosteroid therapy where indicated.

*H. influenzae* can be effectively treated with ampicillin or amoxicillin. Tetracycline and trimethoprim-sulfamethoxazole are reasonable alternatives. *S. pneumoniae* is best treated with penicillin, ampicillin, or amoxicillin as first-line therapy. Erythromycin is an effective second-line treatment for this organism. Trimethoprim-sulfamethoxazole is usually effective. Tetracycline may be useful, but there is a significant incidence of resistance. *M. pneumoniae* can be effectively treated with erythromycin, and tetracycline is an effective alternative.

Any recommendation for the duration of oral therapy is necessarily arbitrary and depends on the severity of the clinical problem. A duration of 10–14 days is commonly recommended. Parenteral treatment may be needed in serious infections or when oral treatment is thought inappropriate.

Prophylactic measures such as influenza vaccination and amantidine should be helpful in preventing exacerbations of asthma due to influenza. A pneumococcal vaccine is also available that is effective against 14 common strains of the *Pneumococcus* for at least 5 years in most patients.

## REFERENCES

1.  McIntosh K, Ellis E, Hoffman L, et al: The association of viral and bacterial respiratory infections with exacerbations of wheezing in young asthmatic children. J Pediatr 82:578, 1973
2.  Hudgel D, Langston L, Selner J, et al: Viral and bacterial infections in adults with chronic asthma. Am Rev Respir Dis 120:393, 1979
3.  Minor T, Reed C: Viruses as precipitants of asthmatic attacks in children. JAMA 227:292, 1974
4.  Schwartz JS: Pneumococcal vaccine: Clinical efficacy and effectiveness. Ann Int Med 96:208, 1982
5.  American College of Physicians. Pneumococcal vaccine recommendations. Ann Int Med 96:206, 1982
6.  The Medical Letter: Influenza prevention for 1980–1981. Med Lett 22(91), 1980
7.  Hirsch M, Swartz M: Antiviral agents. New Engl J Med 302:903, 1980
8.  Amantidine. Ann Int Med 92:256, 1980
9.  Barrett-Connor E: The nonvalue of sputum culture in the diagnosis of pneumococcal pneumonia. Am Rev Respir Dis 103:845, 1971
10.  Leeder S: Role of infection in the cause and course of chronic bronchitis and emphysema. J Infect Dis 131:731, 1975
11.  Tager I, Speizer F: Role of infection in chronic bronchitis. New Engl J Med 292:563, 1975
12.  Burrows B, Nevin W: Antibiotic management in patients with chronic bronchitis and emphysema. Ann Int Med 77:993, 1972
13.  Pines A, Paafat H, Greenfield J: Antibiotic regimens in moderately ill patients with purulent exacerbation of chronic bronchitis. Br J Dis Chest 66:107, 1972
14.  Gump DW, Philip C, Forowyth B: Role of infection in chronic bronchitis. Am Rev Respir Dis 113:465, 1976

15.   Paterson I, Petrie G, Crompton C: Chronic bronchitis: Is bacteriologic examination of sputum necessary? Br Med J 2:537, 1978

16.   Nicotra M, Rivera M, Awe R: Antibiotic therapy of acute exacerbations of chronic bronchitis. Ann Int Med 97:18, 1982

17.   Bates J: The role of infection during exacerbations of chronic bronchitis. Ann Int Med 97:130, 1982

18.   Ingold A: Sputum and serum levels of amoxicillin in chronic baterial infections. Br J Dis Chest 69:211, 1975

19.   Pennington J: Penetration of antibiotics into respiratory secretions. Rev Infect Dis 3(1):67, 1981

20.   Davies B, Maesen F, Brombacher P, et al: Twice daily dosage of bacampicillin in chronic bronchitis. Scand J Respir Dis 59:249–256, 1978

21.   Petersdorf R, Featherstone H: New antimicrobial drugs and their value in the treatment of respiratory infections. Am Rev Respir Dis 117:1, 1978

22.   Johnson A, MacArthur C, Chadwick M, et al: Gastrointestinal absorption and sputum penetration of doxycycline. Am Rev Respir Dis 115(4, Part 2):125, 1977

23.   Hughes D: Single-blind comparative trial of trimethoprim-sulfamethoxazole and ampicillin in the treatment of exacerbations of chronic bronchitis. Br Med J 4:470, 1969

24.   Wormser G, Kersch G: Trimethoprim-sulfamethoxazole in the United States. Ann Int Med 91:420, 1979

25.   Moellering R., Swartz M: The newer cephalosporins. New Engl J Med 294:24, 1976

26.   The Medical Letter: Antibiotics in chronic bronchitis. Med Lett 22(16), August 8, 1980

# Part 4

# Management of the Bronchospastic Patient: Nonpharmacologic Interventions

# Patient Education

## PATIENT EDUCATION: AN OVERVIEW

What do we hope to accomplish with patient education? The ultimate goal is, of course, to improve patient health. A more immediate objective is to produce self-reliant patients who can better understand their diseases and therapies. Such patients can more actively participate in the care process and can be expected to comply better with the medical program.

Blackwell,[1] in his report on drug therapy and patient compliance, says that the most important factor in compliance is the understanding that patients have of their illness and of how the treatment is likely to affect its course. Specifically, the educational process will help patients to:

1. Acquire new knowledge and skills. For example, asthmatics will understand their particular provoking factors or will learn how to use inhalers correctly.
2. Actively participate in their health care. Educated patients will be more able to ask the right questions and make accurate judgments regarding their conditions. For asthmatics, this may lead to more appropriate use of medications and emergency care.
3. Become familiar with new habit patterns such as a realistic routine for dust or allergen avoidance.
4. Achieve an appropriate attitude. Well-informed patients who develop attacks at home will know what to do and will be less likely to panic.

There is not much scientific data substantiating the effectiveness of patient education, probably because the many variables make it difficult to design an adequately controlled study. Those studies that have been done suggest the following beneficial effects: (1) hospitalizations are fewer and shorter, and thus hospital costs are decreased, (2) patients make fewer unnecessary office visits and phone calls, and (3) improved patient compliance reduces emergency room visits.

The Center for Health Promotion of the American Hospital Association publishes a bibliography listing those studies demonstrating the effectiveness of patient education programs.

One report[2] that specifically studied asthmatic patients, was designed to show whether education can decrease health care costs. Asthmatic patients were randomly assigned to control and treatment groups. The treatment subjects attended professionally led group discussions concerning the causes of asthma. Special emphasis was placed on factors that were under the control of the patient such as environmental allergens and ways to avoid them, as well as medications used prophylactically and during an attack. After 4 months, the experimental patients had significantly fewer emergency room visits.

## PATIENT EDUCATION: A PROGRAM FOR THE ASTHMATIC

Patients need to learn about the disease process and their medication or treatment plan. The remainder of this chapter focuses on an asthma educational program that can be tailored to the individual patient with emphasis on those aspects that are most important and easily implemented.

On being instructed about the disease process, the patients are expected to:

1. Define the term "asthma"
2. Explain the basic mechanism of bronchospasm
3. Define the term "provoking factor"
4. Identify their provoking factors
5. Identify appropriate preventive measures for those provoking factors

We try to keep the explanations quite basic. For example, the mechanism of bronchospasm could be explained as simply the contraction of the muscles surrounding the bronchial tubes.

This first group of objectives covers general information on asthma as well as the specifics of the disease process in an individual patient. The general information pertains to all asthmatics and thus lends itself to an audiovisual presentation. A number of suitable cassette or slide-tape instructional programs are available commercially. When audiovisual programs are not feasible, pamphlets on asthma may be of use. Several sources of written materials are listed at the end of this chapter. Many drug manufacturers distribute this type of information as well.

The practitioner would be wise to carefully review the content of any commercial program or pamphlet before buying it. Sometimes the needs of a particular medical practice will not be satisfied by any of the available material and the physician will have to develop personalized teaching aids.

Individualized instruction on the disease process is more difficult with audiovisuals. However, interactive video systems* are being developed that are aimed at creating a patient lesson plan that includes only those provoking factors, preventive measures, and medications relevant to a particular patient. Of course, the traditional teaching methods of one-to-one and group instruction are also useful ways of accomplishing these goals.

The second group of teaching objectives is predominantly concerned with the medication and treatment plan. Patients are expected to:

1. Identify their medications
2. Explain the action of each medication
3. Correctly demonstrate the usage of inhaled or injectable medications
4. Review their individual medication dosage schedules with 100% accuracy
5. Describe those measures to be used at home to treat a mild asthma attack
6. State the guidelines for determining when to seek emergency care

---

*Primarius, 4186 J Sorrento Valley Blvd., San Diego, CA.

Several approaches are needed in order to accomplish these objectives. A certain amount of one-to-one instruction is essential. Written materials are also important, but only as a means of review or reinforcement. Demonstration inhalers containing only inactive substances are a helpful aid to practical instruction.

Useful written materials might include:

1.  Asthma drug information sheets (Fig. 17-1). One sheet is used for each group of drugs and would include the drug's name, dosage and schedule, actions, and common side effects. Suggested groups of drugs would include:

    Antihistamines
    Antihistamines and decongestants-combined
    Bronchodilators—inhaled
    Bronchodilators—oral
    Cromolyn—inhaled
    Steroids—inhaled
    Steroids—intranasal
    Steroids—oral

2.  Medication schedules (Fig. 17-2). These schedules can be designed in a variety of ways and are especially helpful for the elderly or those on a large number of medications with varying instructions.

3.  Procedural instructions (Fig. 17-3a, 17-3b). Written, step-by-step guidelines are essential for continued reinforcement of correct techniques. Sometimes it is helpful to include product and technique information on a single page.

Written materials are important as a means of review and reinforcement but are seldom adequate as the sole or primary method of instruction. Obviously, information on medications needs to be easily read and understood by the patient. To be of maximum benefit, all such materials should be reviewed with the patient in order to prevent misunderstanding. Instruction should be reiterated personally or through other teaching aids.

Demonstration, and more importantly, a successful return demonstration by the patient are crucial components of any technical or procedural instruction. Teaching aids, such as placebo inhalers, are available from drug manufacturers and provide a safe means of "practicing" until correct technique is achieved.

Medication instruction deserves special emphasis because it has been shown that even well-educated patients sometimes comply poorly with medication schedules. Two surveys on the use of aerosol inhalers indicate that many patients use these products inappropriately. One author[3] found that 47% of patients surveyed used an incorrect technique, whereas Epstein[4] reported that only 10.8% of patients in his study group correctly performed all the maneuvers recommended for administration.

All the patients involved in these studies had received some prior instruction in inhaler use; in one study[3] all but four patients had received this instruction from physicians.

Marks,[5] in his study on prophylactic drugs used in asthma management, states that improper instruction in the use of the Spinhaler (Fisons Corporation, Bedford, MA) is probably a major cause of patients discontinuing cromolyn inhalations rather than ineffectiveness of the drug. The development of oral candidiasis in patients using beclomethasone aerosol may also be related to improper technique.[6] If the inhaler is used incorrectly, much of the drug may be deposited in the oral pharynx.

Patient
Education

Scripps Clinic
and Research Foundation

INHALED CROMOLYN POWDER OR SOLUTION

Trade Name: ____________________

Dosage: ____________________

____________________

Use a nebulizer to inhale Cromolyn Solution.
Use a Spinhaler to inhale the powder. Rinse mouth after use if you find the taste unpleasant.

Action: When inhaled, Cromolyn combines with specialized cells to interfere with the release of allergic chemicals. This drug works by preventing asthma so must be used:

--- 15-20 minutes before exercise or exposure to allergens.

--- on a regular basis as your physician ordered.

Possible Side Effects: Cromolyn powder should not be used during active asthma since it may stimulate coughing and wheezing. Skin rashes occur rarely.

For additional information see your pharmacist.
1/83

**Fig. 17-1.** Drug information sheet.

SCRIPPS CLINIC AND RESEARCH FOUNDATION

MEDICATION SCHEDULE

NAME

PHYSICIAN

| DATE | MEDICATION | AMOUNT | TIMES | SPECIAL INSTRUCTIONS |
|------|------------|--------|-------|----------------------|
|      |            |        |       |                      |
|      |            |        |       |                      |
|      |            |        |       |                      |

**Fig. 17-2.** Medication schedule.

129

---

Patient
Education

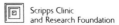 Scripps Clinic
and Research Foundation

**DIVISION OF ALLERGY & IMMUNOLOGY**

---

INHALED STEROIDS


CHEMICAL NAME:   BECLOMETHASONE

TRADE NAME:      VANCERIL

                 BECLOVENT


HOW THE DRUG WORKS

FREON PROPELLENT DELIVERS THE STEROID MOLECULES INTO THE LUNGS
WHERE THEY PROMOTE OPENING OF THE BRONCHIAL TUBES.  THIS DRUG
WORKS BY PREVENTING ASTHMA SYMPTOMS SO IT MUST BE TAKEN REGULARLY
2 TO 4 TIMES A DAY, AS YOUR PHYSICIAN ORDERS.

BECAUSE THIS IS A PREVENTIVE MEDICATION, IT WILL NOT PROVIDE
IMMEDIATE RELIEF DURING AN ASTHMA ATTACK.


DOSAGE

USUAL TREATMENT PROGRAMS MIGHT BE 2 INHALATIONS 2 TO 4 TIMES A
DAY.


SIDE EFFECTS

COUGHING OCCURS RARELY DUE TO THE FREON PROPELLENT.  YEAST (CANDIDA)
GROWS IN THE MOUTH AND THROAT IN 10% OF USERS AND CAN CAUSE SORE
THROAT OR TONGUE.  ALWAYS RINSE YOUR MOUTH WITH WATER OR MOUTHWASH
AFTER USING THE DRUG TO HELP PREVENT THIS PROBLEM.

IF YOU DEVELOP PERSISTEN THROAT PAIN WHILE TAKING THE MEDICATION,
CONTACT YOUR PHYSICIAN.

**Fig. 17-3.**   Combined product and technique information.

Patients need to have a basic understanding of their asthma medications before they leave the physician's office. It is important that the patient understand, how to take the medication and also what can be reasonably expected from use of the drug. As an example, cromolyn may leave an unpleasant taste in the mouth. The patient can be warned about this and assured that rinsing the mouth following a dose will not diminish the drug's effectiveness.

Another major source of confusion for the asthmatic results from the three types of inhaled drug used to treat the disease: bronchodilators, beclomethasone, and cromolyn. Patients will usually assume that all inhaled drugs are equivalent and thus may abandon beclomethasone or cromolyn when it does not provide the prompt relief they have experienced with a bronchodilator. Therefore, patients must understand not only what the effect is but also when it is likely to occur. It is important that the asthmatic be aware of the distinction between prophylactic drugs and those used for immediate relief of symptoms.

We suggest the following approach for teaching inhaler technique. Similar methods

INSTRUCTIONS FOR THE ORAL USE OF INHALERS

1) ASSEMBLE THE INHALER

2) SHAKE THE INHALER WELL

3) PLACE THE MOUTHPIECE IN YOUR MOUTH (JUST PAST YOUR FRONT TEETH) DO NOT CLOSE YOUR LIPS

4) EXHALE COMPLETELY

5) BEGIN TO INHALE AND IMMEDIATELY PRESS DOWN FIRMLY ON THE CAR-TRIDGE.

6) CONTINUE TO INHALE UNTIL YOUR LUNGS ARE COMPLETELY FULL

7) HOLD YOUR BREATH FOR AT LEAST 5 SECONDS (LONGER IF POSSIBLE)

8) EXHALE SLOWLY

IF YOUR PHYSICIAN HAS ORDERED A SECOND INHALATION, WAIT 2 TO 5 MINUTES, THEN REPEAT THE PROCEDURE.

AN EASY METHOD OF ESTIMATING THE AMOUNT OF MEDICATION THAT IS LEFT IN YOUR INHALER IS SHOWN IN THE DIAGRAM. PLACE THE CANISTER IN A BOWL OF WATER AND COMPARE ITS POSITION WITH THE DIAGRAM. WHEN THE CANISTER IS IN THE ¼ FULL POSITION, REFILL YOUR PRESCRIPTION.

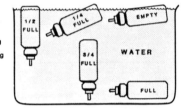

Full: 200 puffs

3/4 Full: approx. 150 puffs remaining

1/2 Full: approx. 100 puffs remaining

1/4 Full: approx. 50 puffs remaining

CARE OF THE INHALER

CLEAN THE MOUTHPIECE AND CAP REGULARLY. USE A COTTONBALL SOAKED IN ALCOHOL AND BE SURE TO REACH ALL THE CREVICES INSIDE THE MOUTH-PIECE.

5/82

**Fig. 17-3.** Continued

could be used to instruct patients in self-injection:

1.  A careful explanation. This is best done either personally or through the use of an audiovisual presentation.
2.  A demonstration and a return demonstration by the patient.
3.  Take-home written instructions for review and reinforcement.
4.  A periodic review at subsequent office visits.

Allergy Foundation of America
801 Second Avenue
New York, NY 10017
(212) 867-8875

American Lung Association
Local Chapter

Cystic Fibrosis Foundation
Local Chapter

National Institute of Allergy
and Infection Disease (NIAID)
Bethesda, MD 20205
(301) 496-5717

## REFERENCES

1. Blackwell B: New Engl J Med 289:249–252, 1973
2. Avery CH, Green LW, Kreider S: Testimony, President's Committee on Health Education, Pittsburgh, PA, 1972
3. Shim C, Williams MH: Am J Med, 69:891–894, 1980
4. Epstein SW, Manning CPR, Ashley MJ, et al: CMA J 120:813–816, 1979
5. Marks MB: Ann Allergy 43:19–23, 1979
6. Imbeau SA, Geller M: JAMA 240:1260–1262, 1978

## SUGGESTED READINGS

Currie BF, Renner JH: Postgrad Med, 657:177–180, 1979
Gillum RF: J Natl Med Assoc 66:156–159, 1974
Maiman LA, Green LW, Gibson, G, et al:
    JAMA, 241:1919–1922, 1979
Somers AR: The Internist, October 3–7, 1977

# 18

RONALD A. SIMON

# Environmental Control and Dust Abatement

The best method of treating asthma, where it is applicable, is to identify and avoid the provoking factors. This is expecially important for asthma provoked by IgE-mediated mechanisms (i.e., allergic or extrinsic asthma). Often the patient has learned to recognize the asthma-causing substances and has taken steps to avoid them before consulting the physician. The allergist's role is to confirm that the patient's observation is valid. Sometimes the history alone is sufficient, and at other times cutaneous tests for immediate hypersensitivity are used to identify an avoidable cause of immediate hypersensitivity. Occasionally, a provocative inhalation challenge, under controlled conditions, is necessary to establish the sensitivity. The role of skin testing and bronchial provocation challenges in the evaluation of the bronchospastic patient has been reviewed in other chapters.

If the bronchospasm develops insidiously or if it is continuous, the problem is more difficult. In such patients, if allergy is playing a role, the responsible substance probably is something the patient is exposed to frequently. Typical examples are house dust, mites, feather pillows, pets, and occupational antigens. It may then be helpful to do a careful history, including an environmental survey or even to have the patient keep a diary listing activities, places visited, and the circumstances in which the asthma attacks occurred or did not occur. Home visits by a knowledgeable professional such as a physician, social worker, office nurse, allergy fellow, or visiting nurse can be very helpful. Patients simply may not recognize certain allergens, may not be able to detect musty odors, or may not think of unusual sources of exposure to allergens.

Most allergists will advise against moving to another part of the country. There will be little beneficial effect if the allergic asthmatic patient continues to sleep on a feather pillow in the same dusty bedroom with a pet nearby.

Meteorologic factors, such as changes in temperature, humidity, barometric pressure, and wind currents can also contribute to an exacerbation of asthma, as do nonspecific environmental irritants, including tobacco smoke, air pollution, aerosol deodorants, air fresheners, perfumes, cleaning compounds, soaps, soot and so on. In fact, an exacerbation of asthma is much more likely to be triggered by one of these factors than by allergens acting through IgE-mediated immediate hypersensitivity mechanisms. The inhaled substances within the home most likely to provoke IgE-mediated asthma include animal danders, house dust, mites, feathers, and indoor mold spores. House dust is ubiquitous, but the most troublesome exposure is usually at night while asthmatics are asleep with their heads buried in dust-laden pillows, mattresses, and blankets for hours on end. For our house-dust-sensitive patients, we recommend use of a vinyl mattress cover that completely encloses the mattress and ziplocks shut. A waterbed also eliminates mattress dust.

Feather pillows should be avoided by asthmatics sensitive to dust and feathers because they tend to decompose into dust before they are replaced. Foam rubber pillows also decompose into dust, and when they are exposed to moisture from perspiration, they become a breeding ground for mold spores. Furry pets should be kept outside the house, even with asthmatics who are not sensitive to danders, because shed hair and the particles of dust and pollen trapped by the fur may act as specific or nonspecific irritants.

Since patients usually spend at least one-third of their time in the bedroom, environmental control measures should be concentrated there. The following are suggestions for control of the bedroom environment, but it should be remembered that the strictness of the control measures should be appropriate for the severity of the symptoms.

Pillows and blankets should be made of synthetic material such as dacron polyester. They should be washed monthly and replaced yearly. Also, the mattress should be completely enclosed in plastic covers, or a waterbed can be used. The bedroom should be cleaned weekly with a damp cloth and the patient should stay out of the room while it is cleaned and for a few hours after. Everything in the room should be dustproof and washable with the use of plain furniture, synthetic or cotton rugs (if any), and synthetic lightweight curtains. Vacuuming should be kept to a minimum because it stirs up dust.

The patient should be encouraged to spend as much time as possible in this room, but the rest of the house must also receive attention if used to any extent. The following steps should be taken to control the environment:

1.  No smoking in the house.
2.  No strong odors, especially perfumes, aerosols, or sprays.
3.  Use an exhaust fan in the kitchen while cooking.
4.  No pets permitted in the house.
5.  House temperature approximately 65°–70°F and relative humidity 30%–50%.
6.  The patient allergic to house dust should stay out of the house during and for several hours after vacuuming.
7.  The patient should not use upholstered furniture or feather pillows.
8.  Washable scattered rugs are preferred, or synthetic rug materials and rubberized rug pads should be used.

The mite *dermatophagoides farinae* (United States) or *pteronyssinus* (Europe) has been shown to be an important antigen in housedust that can provoke asthma symptoms. Many of the suggestions made for house-dust avoidance are effective in reducing mite exposure. Mites thrive on warm, moist air, and thus measures that reduce mold spores in the house will also be effective against house dust.

Molds are nonpathogenic fungi that grow indoors in damp areas such as bathrooms and kitchens. They can also grow in the soil and drainage pans of overwatered houseplants. The growth of mold spores can usually be controlled by proper ventilation, dehumidifiers, and avoiding overwatering of houseplants. Bathroom and kitchen tiles can be scrubbed with a commercial disinfectant. Occasionally, fungicides and trioxymethylkene may be necessary. These can be placed on the floor in an open jar.

There have been some recent reports of immediate hypersensitivity to cockroach antigen. In one study subjects with specific antibodies developed bronchospasm when they inhaled aerosolized cockroach antigen. However, it is not known whether this antigen contributes significantly to asthmatic attacks occurring in the home environment.

In the kitchen, the use of lids on pots and of exhaust fans help to control odors. High-efficiency particulate air filter (HEPA) systems and activated charcoal filters also help to eliminate some odors.

Existing heating systems seldom need modification, but if one is installing a new system, it is worth considering radiant or baseboard heating. There is controversy about whether air conditioning is helpful in controlling allergic respiratory diseases. Although central units will decrease pollen counts during the day, there is little additional benefit from window units in bedrooms since during the nighttime hours, even without filtration, patients only receive 8% of the daily pollen exposure. Most window units do little more than cool the air since their filter systems are ineffective. The unit must be set up to recirculate the indoor room air in order to prevent exposure from outdoor pollens and mold spores, and obviously they accomplish nothing to reduce housedust, mites, and indoor molds.

HEPA filters have been shown to remove more than 99% of particles larger than $0.3\text{-}\mu m$ in diameter. Sometimes one can combine the HEPA filter with a laminar flow device. These can be purchased as room or central units.

Electrostatic air cleaners are inefficient relative to HEPA filters. When homes with the same relative humidity were compared, those with electrostatic air cleaners in forced-air systems had only 16% less contamination than those without the device. Electrostatic air cleaners should not be used as room units because they emit ozone gas.

Humidifiers can be useful in providing additional comfort for some asthmatic subjects. There are many different types and models available that have complex differences, advantages, and disadvantages too numerous to cover in this chapter. The most important fact to remember about humidifiers is that contaminated console and central humidifiers have been shown to cause hypersensitivity pneumonitis. There is a direct relationship between the number of fungus spores in the air and the ambient humidity; thus these units must be fastidiously cleaned.

## SUGGESTED READINGS

Mansmann NC Jr: Environmental control, in Middleton EL, Reed CC, Ellis ER (Eds): Allergy Principles and Practices, St. Louis, Mosby, 1978

Mathison DA, Stevenson DD, Simon RA: Asthma and the home environment (editorial). Ann Int Med 97:128–129, 1982

WALTER L. JENSEN
BRUCE W. ARMSTRONG JR.

# 19

## Aerosol Therapy and Humidification

Aerosol therapy is commonly employed to administer medications to the bronchospastic patient. When delivered in this way, sympathomimetic agents are rapidly effective and require smaller doses than those required by the oral route, reducing the problem of unwanted side effects. When corticosteroids are given by aerosol inhalation, the serious systemic side effects of these agents can be largely avoided. Aerosol inhalation is also the route of administration of cromolyn and of ipratropium, an anticholinergic agent that may soon be available in this country. These agents are described in the appropriate chapters, but in this section we wish to discuss some general aspects of aerosol therapy.

### AEROSOLS

An important parameter used in characterizing therapeutic aerosols is the mass median aerodynamic diameter (MMAD). Fifty percent of the total mass in an aerosol is found in particles whose diameters are smaller or larger than the MMAD. Most of the mass of an aerosol is contained in the larger particles, which thus carry the bulk of the therapeutic agent. The propellant-powered metered-dose inhalers in common use have mass median aerodynamic diameters of 2.6–4.8 $\mu$m, a size small enough to be carried down the lower respiratory tract with the inspired air.[1] Hand-bulb nebulizers produce particles with larger mass median diameters that have a greater tendency to be deposited in the tubing or on the oropharynx. At best, the therapeutic effect is delayed and a larger total dose is often given in order to attain an adequate early therapeutic effect. The larger particles are absorbed more slowly from the pharynx and upper respiratory tract or, when swallowed, from the gastrointestinal (GI) tract, potentially increasing the side effects of the medication. Therefore, we favor the metered dose inhaler for most ambulatory patients. There are some patients, however, who cannot efficiently coordinate their inspiration with actuation of the metered-dose inhaler.

If the mouthpiece is inserted directly into the mouth, a large fraction of the drug is lost because of direct impaction of particles on the tongue and oropharynx before they reach the airways. Unwanted cardiac effects may develop due to absorption of adrenergic agonists through the oropharyngeal mucosa. The deposition of insoluble corticosteroids in the mouth can increase the risk of oropharyngeal candidiasis.

Recently[2-6] some changes in the design of metered-dose inhalers have been recommended in order to make them easier to use and to reduce the problem of impaction loss on the oropharyngeal mucosa. Tubular spacers of different sizes and shapes can be interposed between the jet mechanism and the mouth to ensure that the drug remains suspended in the system for several seconds. Therefore, precise timing of activation of the inhaler at a point of high inspiratory flow is less critical. In addition, the larger particles tend to be deposited on the walls of the tube rather than in the oropharynx. Therefore, a larger fraction of the total dose of the medication ultimately absorbed is delivered to the lower respiratory tract. This should improve the balance between therapeutic effects and systemic side effects.

Sackner et al.[3] have devised a method to evaluate such accessories to a metered dose delivery system. A preinflated, collapsible, plastic reservoir contains a fixed volume (500, 1000, or 1500 ml) and has a fitting to accommodate the metered-dose inhaler. A sound monitoring device emits a noise if inspiratory flow exceeds the desired rate. The inhaler is actuated into the reservoir from which the patient inhales. Aerosol loss by impaction occurs largely within the reservoir bag, not on the patient's oropharyngeal mucosa. In initial studies in bronchitis, 90% retention of aerosols of MMAD 4 $\mu$m occurred within two breaths.

Such reservoir systems would be too bulky for the ambulatory bronchospastic patient, but appropriately designed spacers should provide most of the same advantages with a device that could be carried in a pocket or a handbag. There is no such apparatus in the market at present, but they can be expected to appear in the near future. Most of the above principles can be effectively applied if the patient is properly instructed on the use of the standard metered-dose inhaler.[2] The instruction should be repeated until it is evident that the patient has learned the correct technique. The following points need to be emphasized in using meterd-dose inhalers (MDI).

1. Hold the MDI 4 cm from the wide-open mouth.
2. Exhale completely.
3. Actuate the MDI at the beginning of inspiration.
4. Inspire slowly over 5–6 seconds, drawing the mist deeply into the lungs.
5. Avoid exhaling for approximately 10 seconds.

Dolovich et al.[6] found that if the metered-dose inhaler was held 4 cm from the wide-open mouth, 12% of the total dose was delivered to the lungs. This dose is similar to that obtained when delivery was by a 10-cm extension tube or a 25-cm pear-shaped flask attached to the metered-dose inhaler. In those patients who continued to have difficulty in coordinating the activation of the inhaler with inspiration of the aerosol, spacers may prove advantageous. Spacers attached to steroid inhalers may play an important role in reducing the problem of oral candidiasis.

Another factor influencing the delivery of medication to the lower respiratory tract is the lung volume at the instant when the metered-dose inhaler is actuated. Nebulized terbutaline delivered at the total lung capacity (TLC) showed no bronchodilator effect, whereas the drug inhaled at various lung volumes between the residual volume and 20% below the TLC produced effective bronchodilatation.[2]

## HUMIDIFICATION

Humidity is a term used to describe the water vapor content of gases. Air in the lower respiratory tract is fully saturated at 37°C body temperature through the normal humidification mechanism of the nose. In the bronchospastic patient, incompletely humidified air may reach the lower respiratory tract because of rapid inspiration through the mouth that bypasses the nasal humidifying mechanism and allows insufficient time for water vapor exchange across the oral and pharyngeal mucosa. When air that is unsaturated with water vapor reaches the lower respiratory tract, there are two undesirable consequences. Water is lost from the mucous secretions in the tracheobroncheal tree, making them more viscous and more difficult to expectorate. In addition, the vaporization of water in the airways results in increased respiratory heat loss, which can stimulate bronchospasm.[7] Therefore, in treating an acute asthmatic attack it is important to ensure effective humidification of the inspired air. This is mainly a consideration in the hospitalized patient, but the same principles apply in managing the problem bronchospastic patient at home.

Two types of humidifiers are frequently employed. When oxygen is delivered through nasal prongs or a face mask, the addition of water vapor by use of a simple bubble humidifier has been recommended.[8] In this device, oxygen is directed below the water surface, creating bubbles that return to the top. The humidified oxygen is then carried through plastic tubing and nasal prongs to the patient. Although this is the common practice, it has been shown that bubble nebulizers are inefficient and are probably unnecessary when low-flow oxygen is administered through the nose. They certainly do add significantly to the cost of giving oxygen to the hospitalized patient.

A heated humidifier, usually of the cascade type, is required when the bronchospastic patient has been intubated or has received a tracheostomy. This humidifier produces the large volume of heated, fully saturated water vapor needed to help prevent desiccation of bronchial secretions. In management of a patient placed on a ventilator that bypasses the humidifying action of the nose, we advise that a well-functioning heated humidifier be operating in the circuit. Without such a device, mucociliary clearance rates will rapidly slow and bronchial secretions will inspissate.

## REFERENCES

1. Hiller C, Mazumder MR, Wilson D, et al: Aerodynamic size distribution of metered-dose bronchodilator aerosols. Am Rev Respir Dis 118:311–317, 1978
2. Newman DP, Pavia D, Clarke SW: Simple instructions for using pressurized aerosol bronchodilator. J Roy Soc Med 73:776–779, 1980
3. Sackner MA, Brown LK, Kim CS: Basis of an improved metered aerosol delivery system. Chest 80 (suppl): 915–918, 1981
4. Bloomfield P, Cromptom GK, Winsey NJP: A tube spacer to improve inhalation of drugs from pressurized aerosols. Br Med J 2:1479, 1979
5. Corr D, Dolovich MB, McCormack D, et al: The aerochamber: A new demand-inhalation device for delivery of aerosolized drugs (abstr). Am Rev Respir Dis 121:123, 1980
6. Dolovich M, Ruffin RE, Roberts R, et al: Optimal delivery of aerosols from metered dose-inhalers. Chest 80 (suppl): 911–915, 1981
7. McFadden ER Jr, Ingram RH Jr: Exercise-induced asthma: Observations on the initiating stimulus. New Engl J Med 301:763–769, 1979
8. McPherson SP: Humidifiers and nebulizers. In Respiratory Therapy Equipment, St. Louis, Mosby, 1981, Chapter 4, pp 100–141.

# Psychological Factors and
# Their Management

There are few illnesses in which psychological factors are so clearly prominent, so poorly understood, and so frequently inadequately managed as bronchial asthma. There are few medical conditions in which awareness of and attention to psychological factors is of greater consequence to the success of a total management program.

Despite decades of research into the relationship between emotional and psychological factors and asthma, the subject remains both clouded and controversial. This is true in part because of the nature of asthma itself, which is a disease with many etiologies and varying psychological manifestations. Most physicians dealing with asthmatic patients are aware that emotional factors can be important in triggering symptoms in some of their patients, but pschological components rarely, if ever, represent the major or sole provoking factor.

Even when emotional upsets are identified as contributory, it is easy to ignore them in favor of attending to hypersensitivity, infection, exercise, or other more easily defined precipitants. Frequently, neither physicians nor patients feel comfortable in dealing with the emotional aspects of disease.

The etiology of asthma is still incompletely understood, even though much is known about the pathogenesis of the symptoms of the disease. The currently recognized immunologic and nonimmunologic mechanisms account for only a minority of all asthmatic patients. It is difficult to define clearly the role of psychological factors in a disease that is so incompletely understood.

To complicate matters even further, many psychologists and psychiatrists for years promulgated the incorrect theory that asthma was due to an intense emotional reaction. This influential formulation, first described by two psychiatrists, French and Alexander,[1] led to decades of nonproductive theorizing and research.

## HISTORICAL PERSPECTIVE

The basic premise outlined by French and Alexander greatly influenced psychological theories regarding asthma, and that influence continued for at least 25 years. Much of the large body of psychological research on asthma was generated by efforts to support or to disprove their hypotheses. Today these ideas of 40 years ago seem dated, even amusing, and are generally out of the mainstream of current medical and psychological theories.

Certain views regarding asthma that derive directly from the assumptions inherent in the early work of French and Alexander have attained the status of psychological myth and are still very prevalent in popular, even in some professional, theories. One such myth is that there is a global personality pattern peculiar to asthma or that there are particular personality characteristics associated with asthma. Another myth is that children with asthma experience abnormal relationships with their mothers.

The very real implication of these assumptions is that persons with asthma are in some way psychologically abnormal and that this abnormality is related in some way to the genesis and maintenance of their illness. Such views are clearly fallacious, but they remain widespread despite much contrary evidence and the absence of supporting evidence.

## CURRENT VIEWS

There is no convincing evidence of an asthmatic personality or even of significant specific personality correlates of asthma. Recent comprehensive views on this subject suggest that the degree to which the asthmatic patients differ from "normal" controls is a function of the reliability and validity of the instruments used in the assessment. When more reliable and valid instruments are used, the alleged differences between asthmatics and other groups disappear.

A recent trend has been to compare asthmatic patients to persons with other kinds of chronic illness. Tests evaluating personality disturbances in chronic disease show that the severity of chronic illness is a much more important variable than the specific condition.

The more accurate view, consistent with current medical theory and data concerning asthma, is that there are two ways in which psychological factors interact with asthma. First, psychological and behavioral problems frequently result from the patient's continuing struggles with a disease that interferes with breathing. Such disturbances are not different in kind or intensity than those that result from any chronic illness. Second, in some individuals with asthma, psychological influences such as stress or intense emotional reactions may influence the frequency or intensity of episodes of bronchospastic attacks.

## ASTHMA AS A CHRONIC ILLNESS

What is true is that patients with asthma, like those with any chronic disabling disease, sometimes experience negative affect states such as depression, anxiety, or irritability. Persons with chronic illness also experience feelings of impotence and anger that are poorly expressed because of their enforced dependence on others. The severity of these psychological symptoms depends on many factors, such as the duration of the asthma, how successfully the patient had adapted to it, the degree to which it disrupts normal activity, and to what extent it affects interpersonal relationships, to name only a few.

For the person with asthma, such affective states—which might be considered the expected rather than the pathologic response to chronic illness—may significantly influence the management of the illness itself. The feelings most implicated in the triggering of asthmatic attacks are anger, excitement, pleasure, anxiety, worry, and depression. These emotional states may cause psychological and biologic changes that may in turn influence asthmatic symptoms.

Like any other disease or symptom, asthma may also acquire handicapping properties through social stigmatization and culturally determined attitudes or values, which may magnify the disability as a result of the physical effects of the disease. Any physical attribute can assume handicapping properties when it is seen as a significant obstacle to the accomplishment of a particular goal. It also may become handicapping not because it imposes actual limitations, but because it interferes with social relationships or is in conflict with an individual's value systems. Such changes in attitudes and maladaptive responses can often be forestalled by appropriate attitudes and early intervention by the physician.

## EMOTIONAL FACTORS

It has been commonly observed by both physicians and patients that asthma attacks are more frequent during periods of emotional stress. This may be true even when other precipitating factors such as hypersensitivity, infection, exercise, or atmospheric changes have been clearly identified.

A number of researchers have attempted to induce asthmatic episodes by exposing patients to emotional stress.[2-4] Their data demonstrate that some but not all patients do respond to emotional challenges with a change in their respiratory patterns or a decrease in expiratory flow rate.

Mathe and Knapp[5] considered the apparent paradox of why sympathetic nervous system arousal should induce or enhance bronchospasm since many asthmatic attacks are successfully treated with beta-adrenergic medications. Their data suggest that an adrenergic defect may be involved in some individuals since some of the asthmatics treated produced less than the normal amounts of epinephrine when challenged by emotional stressors.

An alternative hypothesis is that emotionally triggered asthma may result from the stimulation of vagally mediated epithelial irritant receptors. Thus sudden gasping, yelling, crying, or laughing may induce bronchospasm in the same ways that such responses are induced by cold air, airborne irritants, coughing, or other mechanical means.[6] In a controlled study[7] it was shown that 7 of 12 asthmatics were able to reduce the severity of their attacks after being taught to think calmly about their illnesses before and during asthmatic attacks.

In general, the reasonably well-controlled studies cited above, as well as others, demonstrate a tie between emotion and asthma, but the mechanism of the relationship is not clearly understood. Psychological variables do effect pulmonary function in some asthmatic individuals. In some individuals, emotional factors may affect the clinical course of the asthma as well.

## BEHAVIORAL AND INTERPERSONAL FACTORS

The person with early-onset asthma faces severe psychosocial problems that are shared by the entire family. It is this almost universal fact that led to the incorrect hypothesis that there was something about the relationship between the mother and the asthmatic child that caused the asthma problem.

Although asthma is not caused by a faulty mother–child relationship, the importance of the interactions between mother and child in the management of the condition cannot be denied. If the relationship is psychologically unhealthy, it may contribute to behavior detrimental to successful management. More often, however, the mother–child relationship is basically sound and is a positive factor in treatment. In general, mother–child relationships are no different in families with an asthmatic child than in any family in which a child suffers from a chronic disease.

Chronic illness does impose certain stresses on the family system that may have a disorganizing effect if the system is vulnerable, depending on the severity of the stress. Support of the family system is a significant aspect of a total management program.

Asthmatic children tend to grow up isolated from their peers, and many develop poor self-concepts. Academic and social development may be retarded by social isolation and by time lost from school. Parents and others may overindulge the asthmatic child without understanding the child's difficulties. Sometimes the child's asthma becomes the central focus of the family life, governing activities and decisions, major and minor.

Parents frequently experience a wide range of emotions and frustrations associated with raising a child with this kind of illness, including feelings of helplessness, hopelessness, responsibility, guilt, resentment, and anger. These feelings cannot help but affect the asthmatic child as well as the relationships among all family members.

The asthmatic, in turn, is perfectly capable of learning to manipulate others, including parents, teachers, and physicians, and may use the illness as an excuse for poor performance. Many maladaptive behavior patterns can develop that interfere with individual and family functioning.

Sometimes patients develop conditioned fear responses that are triggered by even the possibility of an attack. This is not surprising since asthma is life-threatening. The emotional upset of parents and of those treating a child with severe asthmatic attacks can increase the fears of the patient. These can be fears of hospitals, fears of treatment, and, of course, fears of death. The side effects of medications may interact with emotions, further complicating the picture.

Adult-onset asthma frequently has profound effects on both the patient and the family because of the life-style changes that are required. Like children, adults may become frightened by the symptoms of the disease or by the side effects of the medications, especially sympathomimetic and corticosteroid drugs. Added responsibilities and the financial cost of treating the asthma impose additional burdens on family members.

Asthma thus is a source of behavioral as well as emotional disruption for both patients and families. The physician must be sensitive to the possibility of this disruption regardless of whether it directly affects the symptoms of the disease. Psychological interventions, to be described in the section on psychological treatment, may help in the management of these problems.

## EVALUTING PSYCHOLOGICAL FACTORS

The history-taking skills required for evaluation of possible psychological factors in the asthmatic patient are no different from those used daily by the physician and consist of creating an atmosphere in which the patient and the family feel free to talk. In this atmosphere the history may be systematically reviewed. The minimal relevant data, described more fully by Purcell and Weiss,[8] include a complete and accurate review of the patient's perceptions of the events related to the onset of asthmatic attacks and the asthma symptoms that are affected when the patient interacts with significant others in different ways.

When it has been determined that psychological factors may in part stimulate asthmatic episodes, it may be helpful to refer the patient for behavioral assessment and management. There is little evidence that conventional psychological tests are useful in evaluating the role of emotional factors in asthma. Behavioral (psychological) assessment can, however, help to determine the antecedent behaviors responsible for triggering or aggravating some asthmatic episodes and also in understanding general adjustment, interpersonal relationships, and intellectual and personality strengths and weaknesses. Armed with this information, physicians may be better prepared to help patients and their families to adjust to the illness.

## PSYCHOLOGICAL TREATMENT

There are several ways of treating psychological factors affecting the asthmatic patient. These include psychotherapy, biofeedback, relaxation training, and behavioral management. Psychological treatment is most successful when initiated early and should be aimed at the modification of behaviors that interfere with optimum medical management and the modification of the patient's attitudes toward the asthma symptoms. The last objective may enable a patient to better manage the social and occupational demands of living with asthma without objectively changing the symptoms.

### Psychotherapy

Although any psychological treatment may be considered psychotherapy, the term most often refers to the treatment of psychological problems through verbal means. Psychotherapy can be on an individual basis, in groups or in a family situation. Depending on the nature of the problem and the theoretical orientation of the therapist, psychotherapy is a professional tool used by psychologists, psychiatrists, social workers, and family therapists. Regardless of theoretical bias or the profession of the therapist, psychotherapy should have the goal of assisting the patient and significant others in managing emotions, solving problems, and learning adaptive behavior patterns.

Due to wide variety of psychological problems faced by people with asthma, as well as the many types of therapy, not all therapies are discussed in this chapter. Instead, four types of therapy most relevant to problems particularly associated with asthma are discussed: relaxation training, systematic desensitization, biofeedback, and behavioral management.

### Relaxation Training

There is a growing body of evidence that muscle relaxation has physiologic effects opposite to those induced by psychological and physical stress.[9,10] Not all patients respond in the same ways; however, a thoroughly relaxed person characteristically shows decreased sympathetic nervous system responsiveness and increased parasympathetic activity. This property of the generalized relaxation response led to its importance in behavior therapy. The theory that muscle relaxation has marked effects on the autonomic nervous system has been supported by considerable neurophysiologic evidence.[11]

A number of investigators, but particularly Alexander and his colleagues,[12-14] have demonstrated that psychological relaxation can result in significant decreases in airway resistance. Relaxation retards the natural increase in resistance that occurs when oral bronchodilators are withheld. It has also been demonstrated that premedication with a placebo leads to a significant reduction in exercise-stimulated bronchospasm.[15]

When asthmatic patients can be expected to benefit from reducing sympathetic nervous system responsiveness, any of a large number of relaxation training techniques can be used. These include various forms of meditation training, progressive relaxation training, autogenic training, and biofeedback-assisted relaxation training. Furthermore, relaxation is an integral part of systematic desensitization, which is a procedure used to desensitize asthmatics who have anxieties or phobias related to asthma or aspects of its treatment.

## Systemic Desensitization

Systemic desensitization is a technique devised by Wolpe[16] to help patients cope with anxiety, fears, or phobias. The patient is exposed to the anxiety-arousing stimuli while a physiologic state of relaxation is induced. The patient is gradually exposed to situations with more and more anxiety-evoking potential but is kept in a state of physiologic relaxation, which is incompatible with fear.

Many asthmatic patients experience fear associated with asthma (asthma "panic") that exacerbates or prolongs the attacks. Even when asthma panic does not directly influence the asthmatic attack, its presence leads to unnecessary physical and psychological discomfort.

Of all the treatments tried for asthma panic, systematic desensitization is by far the most effective. Patients with fears or anxieties related to asthma or to any aspect of its treatment may be expected to benefit from this kind of treatment, which is generally brief and focused.

## Biofeedback

Biofeedback applies the principles of learning to alter physiologic behaviors and responses. Electronic or mechanical equipment or other devices are used to measure the physiologic response and to display it to the patient, conveying continuous information as to how the physiologic response is changing. With this information, coupled with systematic reinforcement procedures and practice, patients can often be taught to alter physiologic responses previously felt to be inaccessible to voluntary control (Fig. 20-1). Biofeedback techniques can be used to teach people to relax tense striate muscles or to control normally involuntary autonomic functions such as skin temperature, heart rate, or blood pressure.

Biofeedback methods have been used to try to teach asthmatic patients to modify and control forced expiratory volume ($FEV_1$), peak expiratory flow rate (PEFR), total respiratory resistance (TRR), or other biologic functions related to pulmonary function, such as breath sounds. Asthmatics could be provided with breath-by-breath analyses of their airway resistance, although the instrumentation is necessarily complex. Vachon and Rich[17] and Feldman[18] have reported consistent but small decreases in respiratory resistance in some patients with the use of such methods.

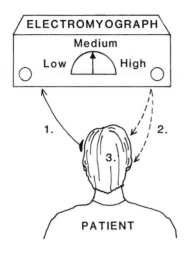

1. Machine records muscle tension from electrodes attached to patient

2. Information recorded is fed back to patient visually or auditorily

3. Using the information provided, the patient learns to change and control muscle tension voluntarily

**Fig. 20-1.**   How biofeedback works, using the electromyographic feedback of muscle tension as an example.

Olton and Noonberg[19] summarized the results of five studies in which asthmatic patients were trained to voluntarily control pulmonary function. They concluded that biofeedback can produce clinically significant results in some patients.

Unfortunately, these studies raise many questions. Their methods require expensive instrumentation, and it has never been demonstrated that this kind of direct biofeedback training produces any better results than the simpler, less expensive use of biofeedback or other methods to teach patients general relaxation techniques. For these reasons the use of biofeedback to teach patients to control pulmonary functions directly should be considered only experimental at this time.

A more effective use of biofeedback is to assist patients in learning general relaxation techniques. This has been more successful, less controversial, and is more widely available. Electromyographic and skin temperature biofeedback are used to help patients learn to decrease muscle tone and sympathetic nervous system activity. These methods, especially when combined with other kinds of training to promote psychological relaxation, can decrease airway resistance in some patients. Studies evaluating the effectiveness of these kinds of treatments have been reviewed recently by Olton and Noonberg.[19]

## Behavioral Management

Behavior modification as a treatment method includes many different techniques, all related to the field of learning. In this context, *behavior* is defined as any activity of an individual that can be observed by another person or measured by an instrument. Biofeedback, relaxation training, and systematic desensitization are special types of behavioral management.

Behavior modification treatment is based on principles of learning theory that are well grounded in an enormous body of experimental data dealing with the relationships between changes in the environment and changes in an individual's responses. The basic principles of behavior modification can be described briefly and with deceptive simplicity.

Since it can be convincingly argued that all human learning is accomplished through classic or operant conditioning, the true complexity becomes readily apparent.

In any chronic disease, including asthma, certain types of behavior can affect the course of the illness, either favorably or unfavorably. The presumption is that if behavior can be altered in a desirable direction, the health of the patient will be improved. Examples of potentially alterable behaviors relevant to asthma might include smoking, medication abuse, or failure to comply with prescribed medical regimens. Other examples include excessive exposure to the emotional precipitants of attacks, inappropriate use of hospitalization, excessive school absence, and the conscious or unconscious precipitation of attacks to manipulate family members or to avoid threatening situations. Behavior modification techniques can be used to manage improper use of inhalation therapy equipment, phobic behaviors that interfere with treatment, attitudes on the part of the patient or family that interfere with management, the adoption of an invalid role, inappropriate social responses, sexual impairment, and medication-induced behavioral changes.

This extensive, but not exhaustive, list includes a large number of problems usually defined as "medical" rather than "behavioral"; however, all of them are responsive to appropriate behavioral analysis and modification. It should be noted that each problem listed implies an alternative behavior beneficial to successful management. The development of these desirable alternative behaviors, rather than the simple elimination of undesirable behaviors, is the ideal goal in behavior modification treatment.

Operant conditioning is the most frequent method of choice in changing human behavior. A behavior is said to be *operant* if the probability of its recurrence is influenced by events that follow it. Any event that follows a response and serves to strengthen that response or increase the likelihood of its reoccurrence is called a *reinforcer*. Different things or events are reinforcing to different people at different times. Food, for example, is reinforcing to the hungry person but not to the one who has just finished eating. Something that may be unpleasant to one person may be reinforcing to another. It is not necessary, although it may be enlightening, to understand why a particular event is reinforcing to an individual. It is important not to have preconceived notions about what things may or may not serve as reinforcers, but to determine this in an objective manner.

Reinforcers can often be identified simply by observing what a person does a lot of. If the patient comes to the hospital frequently, then, by definition, this is a reinforcing activity, and it becomes important to determine what elements in that situation serve as reinforcers. Taking a lot of pills, staying in bed, or visiting physicians frequently can all be reinforcing to some people. If an asthmatic episode is repeatedly followed by an event that is reinforcing to the patient, these attacks may become more frequent or more intense in spite of the obvious aversive characteristics of the attacks.

The point is that behavior can be modified by identifying and selectively manipulating the events that reinforce and maintain the behavior in question. According to this simple principle, with the addition of techniques of shaping and scheduling of reinforcements, it is often possible to alter any of the long list of behaviors previously mentioned.

Three steps are usually involved in operant conditioning of a new response: (1) the existing behavior is carefully analyzed in terms of antecedent events and reinforcements, (2) the baseline occurrence of the desired response is measured, and (3) a potential reinforcer is presented following each occurrence of the response until an increase in the response is clearly demonstrated. Undesired behaviors can be eliminated without the use of aversive or punishing techniques by systematically withdrawing reinforcements for undesirable behaviors and reinforcing desirable alternative behaviors that are incompatible with the response that is being eliminated.

To be effective, reinforcements must be delivered immediately following the behavior to be reinforced, otherwise, one is reinforcing whatever occurred immediately prior to the reinforcement. Once the new behavior occurs regularly, it should be reinforced from time to time so that it is maintained. Even when the response is being reinforced on an intermittent schedule, the reward must be delivered immediately following the desired response.

A couple of difficulties should be apparent at this point. The first is the need for careful analysis in selecting a suitable reinforcer—that is, one that is in fact reinforcing for that individual and is capable of being delivered effectively. This is not an insurmountable problem, but it does require some thoughtful observation and perhaps a little creativity.

The second difficulty is more critical. If the reinforcer, once determined, is to be effective in altering the targeted behavior, it must be delivered consistently and immediately. If one is working with a rat in a Skinner box, there are few problems unless the equipment fails. However, if one is dealing with a human organism, one is likely to have a great deal less control over the multiple situations relevant to that person's life. It is of critical importance that the procedures be carried out consistently in all settings, or in as many settings as one can possibly influence. Therefore, the persons around the patient must be knowledgeable and cooperative in maintaining the program. It is not sufficient to work with patients in a limited setting that has little relevance to their daily lives and ignore family, school, work, and other environments. When a behavior modification program fails, it is most likely that one or the other of these factors have been ignored.

Numerous examples of the applications of behavioral management are available, many of which have been described by Creer.[20] Renne and Creer,[21] for example, used positive reinforcement procedures to teach an asthmatic child to use an intermittent positive-pressure breathing (IPPB) device properly. They rewarded what they identified as correct responses such as eye fixation, facial posturing, and diaphragmatic breathing until the child was using the device properly. As the patient became more and more proficient in using the equipment, less medication was also required.

The systematic withholding of reinforcement (extinction) to reduce an undesirable behavior was used by Neisworth and Moore.[22] They instructed the parents of an asthmatic child to stop providing sympathy and attention for coughing episodes that exceeded what was expected in their child on the basis of the severity of the child's asthma. Withholding of the reinforcements of sympathy and attention produced a dramatic reduction in the number of coughing episodes.

Creer[20] has used the withdrawal of positive reinforcement to manage malingering behaviors in asthmatic children. Each time such a child would be admitted to the hospital, usually when faced with some kind of stress, all the pleasant aspects of hospitalization such as games, books (other than homework), television, and visiting privileges were withheld. In several cases the frequency and duration of hospitalizations decreased markedly. Creer[20] and others have used various kinds of behavioral techniques to increase study time in asthmatic children, to suppress coughing symptoms, to decrease the abuse or misuse of medications, and to decrease behaviors that precipitate asthmatic episodes (e.g., yelling, screaming, hyperventilation, breath-holding).

The applications of behavioral techniques to the management of asthma-related behaviors is almost unlimited. Rehabilitative treatment and management, by definition, focuses on the changing of behaviors in patients and their families. Many asthmatic patients demonstrate a variety of maladaptive behaviors that aggravate their conditions. Although none of these techniques has ever been demonstrated to affect the underlying respiratory processes, they can have profound effects on the patient's adjustment to the symptoms of the disease.

## PERSPECTIVES ON NEW AND FUTURE DEVELOPMENTS

In contrast with traditional thinking, it is now believed that psychological factors are not related to the etiology of asthma. For some patients, however, emotional episodes can trigger or exacerbate asthmatic attacks. Therefore, asthma may be improved, but it cannot be cured by psychological treatments.

Experiments on biofeedback techniques have not demonstrated convincingly a direct influence on lung function except in a few patients. Perhaps in the future there will be improvements in biofeedback or similar methods that will be of more benefit to larger numbers of asthmatic patients.

Biofeedback is, however, an effective technique for teaching some patients to relax. Where relaxation training is a necessary part of treatment, as in the systematic desensitization of fears and phobias associated with asthma, biofeedback can be a helpful adjunct to treatment.

Many asthmatic patients do have problems with fear and anxiety, problems in adhering to medical regimens, and problems with adjustment to living, both in and outside of the family. The techniques of behavior medicine are being used more and more to deal with these consequences of asthma and will be even more widely applied as physicians become more aware of them.

Asthma is a chronic disease, and once the condition is stabilized medically, rehabilitation is important. Rehabilitation is most effective when physicians, patients, families, and behavioral specialists work together as a team to solve the problems created by the patient's illness.

## REFERENCES

1. French TM, Alexander F: Psychogenic factors in bronchial asthma. Psychosom Med Mono 14:2–94, 1941
2. Clarke PS: Effects of emotion and cough on airways obstructions in asthma. Med J Aust 1:535–549, 1970
3. Hill E: Bronchial reactions to selected psychological stimuli and concomitant autonomic activity and asthmatic children. Unpublished doctoral dissertation, State University of New York, Buffalo, 1975
4. Weiss JH, Lyness J, Molk L, et al: Induced respiratory change in asthmatic children. J Psychosom Res 20:115–123, 1976
5. Mathe AA, Knapp PH: Emotional and adrenal reactions to stress in bronchial asthma. Psychosom Med 33:323–338, 1971
6. Gold WM, Kessler GR, Yu DYC: Role of vagus nerves in experimental asthma in allergic dogs. J Appl Physiol 33:719–725, 1972

7. Yorkston NJ, Eckert E, McHugh RB, et al: Bronchial asthma: Improved lung function after behavior modification. Psychosomatics 20:325–331, 1979

8. Purcell K, Weiss JH: In Costello CG (Ed): Symptoms of Physiopathology, New York, Wiley, 1978

9. Benson H: The Relaxation Response. New York, Morrow, 1975

10. Stoyva JM: *In* Beatty, J, Legewie H (Eds): Biofeedback and Behavior, New York, Plenum, 1977

11. Germana J: Central efferent processes and autonomic-behavioral integration. Psychophysiology 6:78–90, 1969

12. Alexander AB: Systematic relaxation and flow rates in asthmatic children: Relationship to emotional precipitants and anxiety. J Psychosom Res 16:405–410, 1972

13. Alexander AB, Miklich DR, Hershkoff H: The immediate effects of systematic relaxation training on peak expiratory flow rates in asthmatic children. Psychosom Med 34:388–394, 1972

14. Alexander AB, Cropp GJA, Chai H: The effects of relaxation training on pulmonary mechanics in children with asthma. J Appl Behav Anal 12:27–35, 1979

15. Godfrey S, Silverman M: Demonstration by placebo response in asthma by means of exercise testing. J Psychosom Res 17:293–297, 1973

16. Wolpe J: Psychotherapy by Reciprocal Inhibition, Stanford, Stanford University Press, 1958

17. Vachon L, Rich ES: Visceral learning in asthma. Psychosom Med 38:122–130, 1976

18. Feldman GM: The effect of biofeedback training on respiratory resistance of asthmatic children. Psychosom Med 38:27–34, 1976

19. Olton DS, Noonberg AR: Biofeedback: Clinical Applications in Behavioral Medicine. Englewood Cliffs, NJ, Prentice-Hall, 1980

20. Creer TL: Asthma Therapy: A Behavioral Health Care System for Respiratory Disorders, New York, Springer, 1970

21. Renne C, Creer TL: The effects of training on the use of inhalation therapy equipment by children with asthma. J Appl Behav Anal 9:1–11, 1976

22. Neisworth JT, Moore F: Operant treatment of asthmatic responding with the parent as therapist. Behav Ther 3:95–101, 1972

Part 5

# Special Problems in Asthma

Michael Schatz
Robert S. Zeiger

# 21

# The Upper Airway and Asthma: Physiological and Clinical Relationships

Asthma and upper airway disease, chiefly of the nose and sinuses, frequently coexist. In one series, 78% of patients with extrinsic asthma had nasal symptoms.[1] In another, 52% of adult asthmatics had abnormal sinus films, which is approximately twice the incidence in the "normal" nonasthmatic population.[2] In a group of 476 infants and children with asthma, abnormal sinus films were found in 62%.[3] Conversely, patients with rhinitis frequently develop asthma. The cumulative prevalence of perennial asthma in hay fever patients is 5%–10%, which is two or three times the normal risk.[1,4] In one series, episodes of asthma occurred in 32% of patients with allergic rhinitis.[1] Similarly, Connell[5] has reported the occurrence of perennial asthma in 30% of patients with eosinophilic nonallergic rhinitis, and 18% of patients with nasal mastocytosis.

There are two main explanations for the frequent coexistence of asthma and upper airway disease. First, the two conditions may result from the same genetic and environmental factors. An inherited atopic tendency and genetic linkage of upper and lower airway end-organ abnormalities as well as similar adverse effects of environmental factors on the entire airway could account for the occurrence of upper and lower airway disease in the same patients. Second, there may be a relationship between upper airway disease and asthma, such that upper airway disease causes or at least exacerbates the asthma. Although there are large gaps in our knowledge in this area, this chapter explores the information relating to the possibility of a mechanistic relationship between upper airway disease and asthma. In addition, this chapter explores the clinical, diagnostic, and therapeutic implications of such a relationship. The reader is referred elsewhere for background information regarding upper airway anatomy and physiology.[6,7]

## THE UPPER AIRWAY AND PULMONARY PATHOPHYSIOLOGY

Abnormal upper airway function could affect pulmonary pathophysiology because of poorly conditioned or filtered air, additional airway resistance, upper airway reflexes affecting the bronchi, or upper airway infections.

## Nasal Obstruction and Pulmonary Obstruction

Nasal obstruction can of itself increase airways resistance. Ogura[8] reported that abnormal pulmonary resistance associated with nasal septal deviation returned to normal 4–6 months following successful surgical treatment in 85% of the cases tested. There have been several studies suggesting that the interaction between the upper respiratory tract and bronchoconstriction results from parasympathetic reflexes. The administration of cold aerosols into the nose caused an increase in pulmonary resistance of asthmatics as measured by a forced oscillation technique. The response occurred even in laryngectomy patients whose upper and lower respiratory systems were not connected.[9] Sulfur dioxide inhalation produces both increased nasal airway resistance and bronchoconstriction. When sulfur dioxide was introduced into the anatomically separated upper airways of cats, there was constriction of the lower airways, suggesting that the bronchoconstriction was caused by a reflex originating in the upper airway. The bronchospasm was blocked by atropine, suggesting that the reflex involved is cholinergic parasympathetic.[10] In contrast to Ogura's data, however, a recent study using xenon-133 pulmonary ventilation scintigraphy showed no evidence of airstreaming or reflex bronchoconstriction in three patients with nasal septal deviation.[11]

## Rhinitis and Bronchospasm

Pulmonary function testing in many patients with rhinitis without clinical asthma has demonstrated obstruction of both large airways[12] and small airways.[13-15] In one study,[15] the abnormal frequency-dependence of compliance and abnormal closing capacity demonstrated during seasonal rhinitis resolved when the patients were retested in the winter after their nasal symptoms had cleared.

In addition to airway obstruction, bronchial hyperreactivity has been demonstrated in patients with rhinitis without clinical asthma. Stevens and Vermiere[16] showed that histamine-induced decreases of $FEV_1$ in rhinitis patients were intermediate between those of control subjects and asthma patients. Similarly, Deal, et al.[17] reported that the decreased $FEV_1$ in response to hyperpnea with cold air in some patients with allergic rhinitis was intermediate between controls and asthmatic patients. Gniazdowski[18] reported greater than a 10% decrease in $FEV_1$ following histamine inhalation in 58% of hay fever patients, 53% of patients with nasal polyps, 22% of patients with nonallergic rhinitis, and only 6%–8% of control populations.

Fish et al.[19] demonstrated that the site of bronchial hyperreactivity in the rhinitis patient may differ from that in the asthmatic. After methacholine challenges, the specific airways conductance decreased in rhinitis patients, whereas both $FEV_1$ and specific conductance fell in patients with asthma. This suggests that asthmatics possess hyperreactivity of both central and peripheral airways whereas nonasthmatic patients with hay fever have hypersensitivity in large central airways only. All these data would be consistent with a cause–effect relationship between rhinitis and bronchial obstruction or hyperreactivity. However, they could also be manifestations of subclinical asthma in these rhinitis patients known to be at increased risk of asthma.

It is of interest that the results of antigen inhalation challenges do not differentiate allergic rhinitis patients from asthma patients.[16,20,21] In studies with ragweed, mite, and grass pollen, pulmonary function abnormalities and bronchodilator responses were qualitatively and quantitatively similar in allergic rhinitis patients without asthma and in patients with allergic asthma, although nonspecific bronchial reactivity was significantly different between the two groups. This has two mechanistic implications: (1) nonspecific bronchial reactivity may be of primary importance in determining whether an allergic patient manifests asthma; and (2) the type of antigen exposure involved in inhalation challenge may be substantially different from that involved in natural environmental exposure.

Pulmonary function abnormalities can be elicited by upper respiratory infections in nonasthmatic patients. Infections with the common cold viruses (especially rhinovirus) and influenza A can be followed by persistent (3–8 weeks) abnormalities of pulmonary function and increased bronchial hyperreactivity.[22] Although these data would be consistent with the concept that the upper airway abnormalities cause the lower airway abnormalities, a direct effect of the viruses on the lower airway cannot be excluded.

## The Upper Airway and Exercise/Cold Air-Induced Bronchospasm

The model of bronchospasm where the data are most suggestive of an important relationship with the upper airway is the bronchospasm induced by exercise and by cold air. Several studies have shown that exercise-induced asthma may be attenuated by nasal breathing.[23-25] Recently Griffin et al.[25] studied exercise-induced asthma with and without nasal breathing while measuring the temperature in the retrotracheal esophagus. They found that the temperature in the esophagus (and presumably the airways) was significantly lower with oral than with nasal breathing, and they demonstrated a linear relationship between the degree of airway cooling and the severity of subsequent bronchoconstriction. Since current concepts of exercise-induced asthma suggest that loss of heat and water from inspired air is important in the pathogenesis,[26] it seems clear that the beneficial effect of nasal breathing is due to the presentation of better conditioned air to the airways of the lower respiratory tract. However, the site at which the cold, dry air stimulates bronchoconstriction is not established.

Several studies have suggested that cold air causes bronchospasm by stimulating upper airway receptors, thus provoking reflex bronchoconstriction, probably through cholinergic pathways. McNally et al.[27] reported that oropharyngeal anesthesia decreased exercise-induced bronchospasm in 4 of 10 patients. Aquilina et al.[28] showed that breathing cold air during exercise causes bronchospasm in nonasthmatic subjects with upper respiratory infections, which may be blocked by atropine or oropharyngeal anesthesia. Enright et al.[29] demonstrated that pretreatment with an aerosol of 4% lidocaine (which blocked cough-and-gag reflexes) blocked exercise-induced bronchospasm in asthmatic subjects. Strauss et al.[30] reported that the application of ice to the buccal mucosa caused bronchoconstriction in asthmatics, preventable by topical anesthesia. Finally, Rodriguez-Martinez et al.[31] were able to prevent cold-air-induced bronchoconstriction in a group of asthmatic children by previous topical anesthesia of the pharynx with 4% lidocaine.

In contrast to the above data, controlled data from McFadden's laboratory[32,33] have been unable to confirm an effect of oropharyngeal or inhaled lidocaine on exercise-induced asthma. These authors cite data showing that cooling of the intrathoracic airways initiates bronchoconstriction and explain that the beneficial effect of nasal breathing is through more efficient conditioning of the inspired air before it reaches the intrathoracic airways.[25] Regardless of the exact mechanism whereby nasal breathing attenuates bronchospasm, this model provides a direct physiologic basis for the hypothesis that improved nasal

**Table 21-1**

**Clinical Classification of Chronic Rhinitis with Etiologic, Diagnostic, and Therapeutic Characteristics**

| Type of Rhinitis | Allergic Rhinitis | Eosinophilic Nonallergic Rhinitis | Nasal Polyps | Rhinitis Medicamentosa | Structural Rhinitis | Primary Vasomotor Instability | Neutrophilic Rhinosinusitis |
|---|---|---|---|---|---|---|---|
| Cause or mechanism | Intranasal IgE-mediated reaction to allergens (usually inhalant) | Nasal mucosal eosinophilic infiltration of unknown etiology | Non-neoplastic fluid-filled mucosal sacks of unknown etiology | Topical or systemic medication affecting nasal autonomic nervous system | Septal abnormalities | Nasal mucosal hyperreactivity due to autonomic nervous imbalance not associated with local nasal disease | Variably virulent chronic or intermittent bacterial infection of posterior nasopharynx or paranasal sinuses |
| Characteristic symptoms | Runny nose, sneezing, eye irritation | Congestion, nose blowing | Congestion, anosmia | Congestion | Unilateral obstruction | Congestion | Postnasal drip, sinus pain |
| Seasonal variation | Seasonal or perennial | Perennial | Perennial | Perennial | Perennial | Perennial | No specific seasonal variation but may be worse in winter |
| Associated factors | Onset age 1–20 or with change in environment, family history of atopy | Onset age 20–40, asthma, aspirin sensitivity | Onset age 20–40, asthma, aspirin sensitivity | Topical decongestant abuse, antihypertensive therapy | Nasal trauma | Hormonal (pregnancy, oral contraceptives, thyroid disorders), systemic autonomic nervous system dysfunction, no identifiable associated factors in some patients | IgA deficiency, hypogammaglobulinemia, cystic fibrosis, immotile cilia syndrome, may follow viral URI, may complicate eosinophilic rhinitis or nasal polyps, may occur without identifiable underlying cause |

| Physical exam, laboratory findings | Nasal smear | Symptomatic therapy | Other therapy |
|---|---|---|---|
| Mucosa pale, positive skin tests, correlating with history | Eosinophils with or without mast cells | Antihistamines, decongestants, topical corticosteroids | Antigen avoidance, immunotherapy |
| Mucosa pale, edematous, negative or coincidentally positive skin test | Eosinophils with or without mast cells | Antihistamines, decongestants, topical corticosteroids, oral corticosteroids (occasionally) | Treat complicating infection |
| Polyps on physical exam | Usually eosinophils with or without mast cells | Antihistamines, decongestants, topical corticosteroids, oral corticosteroids | Treat complicating infection, polypectomy |
| Unremarkable or erythematous mucosa | Normal | Topical corticosteroids for topical decongestant abuse | Discontinue responsible medication |
| Septal abnormality on physical examination | Normal | None | Surgery |
| Turbinate swelling | Normal | Decongestants (oral and intermittent topical), nasal saline | Treat systemic disorder, exercise |
| Sinus films usually (not always) abnormal acutely or chronically, mucopurulent secretions, sinus tenderness, exam may be normal | Neutrophils with or without bacteria | Decongestants (oral and intermittent topical) antihistamines, nasal saline | Antibiotics, sinus surgery |

159

function in a patient with rhinitis and asthma may be beneficial regarding the broncho-spasm.

## UPPER AIRWAY DISEASE AND ASTHMA: CLINICAL IMPLICATIONS

The preceding information does not establish a mechanistic relationship between upper airway disease and asthma in all or even most cases. Combined with clinical observations, however, this knowledge suggests that optimal treatment of upper airway disease in patients with asthma may have beneficial effects on the asthma as well as on the upper airway problem.

Rhinitis and sinusitis are the most common problems encountered in the upper airways of asthmatic patients, and these are discussed in the following section. In addition, one must remember that upper airway obstruction must be considered in the differential diagnosis of asthma in children and adults. Spirometry may be of some assistance in identifying upper airway obstruction,[34] but laryngoscopy or bronchoscopy is generally necessary for making a definitive diagnosis.

Chronic cough is a common problem in both upper airways disease and in asthma. Certain patients with chronic cough and normal pulmonary function tests can be shown by methacholine challenge to have hyperreactive airways (see Chapter 7). In these patients the cough may respond to asthma therapy. Postnasal drip is one of several upper airway causes of chronic cough,[35] and a recent study suggests that postnasal drip or asthma, or the combination of the two accounts for approximately 70% of the cases of chronic cough referred to pulmonary specialists for diagnosis.[36]

## RHINITIS-SINUSITIS AND ASTHMA

### Classification of Chronic Rhinitis-Sinusitis

A clinically useful classification of chronic rhinitis is shown in Table 21-1, but such a classification has several limitations. First, the exact causes of many types of chronic rhinitis are not well understood, and thus the classification must be considered tentative relative to etiologic and pathogenetic implications. Second, several causes of rhinitis may coexist in the same patient, complicating and potentiating each other. Finally, not every patient can be unequivocally assigned to a single diagnostic category, especially on initial evaluation. Nonetheless, such a classification provides a useful framework on which to base an organized diagnostic and therapeutic approach.

### Diagnostic Approach to Chronic Rhinitis-Sinusitis

Assignment to a diagnostic category can generally be made on the basis of the history, limited physical examination, and nasal scraping. The history should identify the following information: (1) the specific symptom complex, (2) the circumstances of onset of the symptoms (e.g., childhood vs adult onset or following infection, trauma, or an environmental change), (3) factors that precipitate symptoms, (4) the seasonal variation of the symptoms, and (5) associated factors (e.g., topical and oral medication usage or coexistent endocrine conditions).

Physical examination of the nose establishes the diagnosis of nasal polyps or septal abnormalities and allows the degree of mechanical obstruction and the nature of nasal secretions to be ascertained. A good view of the middle meatus and middle turbinates is required for complete evaluation of the nose. This may necessitate application of a topical decongestant to shrink obstructing inferior turbinate tissue.

The most useful physical examination technique for examining the sinuses is percussion for tenderness. Transillumination is relatively unreliable, especially for maxillary sinus disease.[37] There may be substantial sinus disease in the absence of abnormal physical findings.[38] To complete the upper airway physical examination in a patient with rhinitis, the eyelids and conjunctiva, the pharynx and tonsils, and the tympanic membranes should be evaluated.

The nasal scraping is used to identify various important mucosal cellular elements. It is obtained and stained as described in Table 21-2. In conjunction with the history and physical examination, the nasal scraping will usually indicate a specific pattern of rhinitis.

**Table 21-2**
**Technique for Performance of Nasal Cytologic Evaluation**

Collection of material

Label a slide with patient's name on frosted end with PENCIL ONLY
Use flexible Rhinoprobe* with plastic tip
Use illuminated nasal speculum
Place the Rhinoprobe* tip into the nose onto inferior tubinate
Gently press Rhinoprobe tip on mucosa of inferior tubinate and move 2-3 mm toward you
Gently press mucosa that is in the level tip in a quick movement, not smeared, onto slide
Immediately place slide in a 95% alcohol solution and leave it there until used for staining

Staining of slides

Preparing three staining dishes and label Wright-Giemsa Stain,* Volu-Sol Buffer,* and Volu-Sol Rinse*
Place slides in staining rack
Place slide rack in stain for exactly 15 seconds
Remove and place rack in buffer for exactly 30 seconds
Remove and place rack in rinse for approximately 4 seconds
Remove and drain rack on absorbent paper and let slides dry with a fanned blow dryer

Microscopic examination

Scan entire slide at low power ( × 100) initially; mast cells, clumps of eosinophils, epithelial cells, and
    goblet cells are easily identified at this power
Observe at × 450 if there is any doubt about a particular cell
Reserve oil immersion screening for identifying bacteria and make it the last examination
    procedure

*Rhinotechnics
P.O. Box 84058
San Diego, CA 92138

Follow-up nasal scrapings after initial therapy are frequently necessary for definition of the total nasal pathology.

Depending on these findings, sinus films, total serum IgE, and allergy skin tests may be considered. Patients with neutrophilic rhinosinusitis, eosinophilic nonallergic rhinitis, and nasal polyps should have sinus films taken to rule out complicating sinus disease. In addition, since infectious sinusitis in patients with asthma may be associated with minimal clinical symptoms or signs,[38] sinus films probably should also be taken for patients with any form of rhinitis associated with substantial asthma. Abnormal sinus films, especially with air-fluid levels or opacification, may indicate complicating sinus infection, although normal sinus films, it seems, do not rule out infection limited to the nasopharynx. Conversely, even without infection there may be mucosal thickening on the sinus radiographs of patients with eosinophilic nonallergic rhinitis or nasal polyps. In some patients, therefore, the total clinical picture and possibly sinus irrigation may be necessary for determining the significance of abnormal sinus films.

Properly performed skin tests identify allergen-specific IgE, (see Chapter 5) which, when correlated with clinical findings, helps to confirm a diagnosis of allergic rhinitis. The finding of a total serum IgE level of greater than 50 IU/ml by paper radioimmunosorbent (PRIST) assay (in conjunction with the remainder of the evaluation) may be a useful screening test for identifying patients who should be referred to allergists for complete allergy testing.[39] However, by itself the total serum IgE level can neither confirm nor exclude a diagnosis of allergic rhinitis. Persons predominantly sensitive to house dust have normal IgE levels.[40] Moreover, most patients with allergic or nonallergic rhinitis associated with asthma will have an elevated serum IgE level.[6]

## Specific Forms of Rhinitis: Diagnostic and Therapeutic Implications

The therapy of the various types of chronic rhinitis is summarized in Table 21-1 and reviewed elsewhere.[6,41,42] Any successful therapy of rhinitis may potentially improve coexisting asthma; however, this section deals with the therapy of those types of rhinitis with established relevance to coexisting asthma. In addition, certain specific diagnostic relationships between the various types of rhinitis and asthma are discussed.

### Allergic Rhinitis

As discussed previously, inhalation challenge does not differentiate patients with allergic asthma from those with allergic rhinitis only. Consequently, antigen inhalation challenge cannot be used to diagnose asthma in an allergic patient.

Antihistamines may be very useful in the treatment of patients with allergic rhinitis. However, many antihistamine package inserts state that antihistamines should not be given to patients with asthma because of the theoretical concern about drying of bronchial secretions. This concern is apparently unfounded since recent studies suggest that there is no adverse effect of antihistamines on patients whose asthma is being appropriately managed.[43]

Johnstone[44] suggested that immunotherapy of allergic rhinitis in children may prevent the subsequent development of asthma. No confirmatory studies have been published, and the great majority of allergic rhinitis patients do not subsequently develop asthma.[1,4] Therefore, we do not believe that the overall data justify immunotherapy of allergic rhinitis solely to prevent asthma.

### Eosinophilic Non-allergic Rhinitis

The etiology of this condition is not known. However, it appears to be frequently associated with frank asthma or at least bronchial hyperreactivity manifest by methacholine sensitivity.[45] In addition, such patients may develop nasal polyps, sinusitis, and the entire aspirin idiosyncracy syndrome.

### Nasal Polyps

Certain authors have suggested that surgical removal of nasal polyps may precipitate or exacerbate coexistent asthma. However, a study of polypectomies in 101 aspirin-triad patients does not confirm this.[46] The asthma at 1 year after compared to 1 year before polypectomy was better in 30 patients, unchanged in 57, and worse in only 14. Postoperative wheezing occurred in 20 patients and was most common in those with active asthma prior to surgery. We conclude that polypectomy should be considered in patients with nasal polyps with or without coexistent asthma when they are not doing well on medical therapy. In patients who have asthma, the asthma must be optimally controlled preoperatively.

### Neutrophilic Rhinosinusitis

The differential diagnosis in patients with sinusitis and lower respiratory disease includes hypogammaglobulinemia, immunodeficiency with hyperimmunoglobulinemia E, cystic fibrosis, and the immotile cilia syndrome. In addition, as noted earlier, asthma and sinus disease frequently coexist in the absence of these conditions.

When asthma coexists with abnormal sinus radiographs, bacterial sinusitis cannot always be confirmed. In fact, Berman et al.[2] reported that sinus aspirates yielded bacterial growth in only 20% of 32 asthmatic patients with abnormal sinus films. Nonetheless, empiric observations suggest that sinus infections may substantially influence asthma in that asthma frequently flares with nasal and/or sinus infections; persistent sinusitis may be a cause of recalcitrance to usual asthma therapy; and substantial improvement in asthma control usually follows appropriate medical or surgical therapy of the sinus disease.[38] Physicians managing asthmatic patients must have a high index of suspicion for complicating sinus infections, especially in those patients not responding well to therapy.

## REFERENCES

1.  Smith JM: In Middleton EL, Reed CE, Ellis EF (Eds): Allergy: Principles and Practice, St. Louis, Mosby, 1978, pp 633–658
2.  Berman SZ, Mathison DA, Stevenson DD, et al: Maxillary sinusitis and bronchial asthma: Correlation of roentgenograms, cultures, and thermograms. J Allergy Clin Immunol 53:311–317, 1974
3.  Kolbar V, Lokar R: Disorders in rhinosinusal regions and asthma in children. Acta Med Yugosl 33:299–305, 1979
4.  Broder I, Higgins MW, Mathews KP, et al: Epidemiology of asthma and allergic rhinitis in a total community, Tecumseh, Michigan. J Allergy Clin Immunol 53:127–138, 1974
5.  Connell JT: In Weiss EF, Segal MS (Eds): Bronchial Asthma: Mechanisms and Therapeutics, Boston, Little, Brown, 1976, pp 481–489
6.  Mygind N: Nasal Allergy, Oxford, Blackwell Scientific Publications, 1978

7. Proctor DF: The upper airways: Nasal physiology and defense of the lungs. Am Rev Respir Dis 115:97–129, 1977

8. Ogura JH: Physiologic relationships of the upper and lower airways. Ann Otolaryngealol 79:495–498, 1970

9. Takagi T, Proctor DF, Salmon S, et al: Effects of cold air and carbon dioxide on nasal air flow resistance. Ann Otol 78:40–48, 1969

10. Nadel JA, Salem H, Tamplin B, et al: Mechanism of bronchoconstriction during inhalation of sulfur dioxide. J Appl Physiol 20:164–167, 1965

11. Silberstein EB, Lewis JT, Quenelle DJ: A study of the physiologic relationship of lower and upper airways with $^{133}$Xe. Ann Otolaryngealol 89:62–64, 1980

12. Fairshter RD, Novey HS, Marcholi LE, et al: Large airway constriction in allergic rhinitis: Response to inhalation of helium-oxygen. J Allergy Clin Immunol 63:39–46, 1979

13. Grossman J, Putnam JS: Small airway obstruction in allergic rhinitis. J Allergy Clin Immunol 55:49–55, 1975

14. Lidington RE, Cotton DS, Graham BL, et al: Peripheral airways obstruction in patients with rhinitis. Ann Allergy 42:28–33, 1979

15. Morgan EJ, Hall DR: Abnormalities of lung function in hay fever. Thorax 31:80–86, 1976

16. Stevens WJ, Vermiere PA: Bronchial responsiveness to histamine and allergen in patients with asthma, rhinitis, cough. Eur J Respir Dis 61:203–213, 1980

17. Deal EC, McFadden ER, Ingram RH, et al: Airway responsiveness to cold air and hyperpnea in normal subjects and in those with hay fever and asthma. Am Rev Respir Dis 121:621–628, 1980

18. Gniazdowski R: Perennial atopic rhinitis as an early stage of bronchial asthma. Acta Otolaryngealol 88:257–267, 1979

19. Fish JE, Rosenthal RR, Batra G, et al: Airway responses to methacholine in allergic and nonallergic subjects. Am Rev Respir Dis 113:579–586, 1976

20. Fish JE, Ankin MG, Kelly JF, et al: Comparison of responses to pollen extract in subjects with allergic asthma and nonasthmatic subjects with allergic rhinitis. J Allergy Clin Immunol 65:154–161, 1980

21. Ahmed T, Fernandez RJ, Wanne A: Airway responses to antigen challenge in allergic rhinitis and allergic asthma. J Allergy Clin Immunol 67:135–145, 1981

22. Hall WJ, Douglas RG: Pulmonary function during and after common respiratory infections. Ann Rev Med 31:233–238, 1980

23. Shturman-Ellstein R, Zeballas RJ, Buckley JM, et al: The beneficial effect of nasal breathing on exercise-induced bronchoconstriction. Am Rev Respir Dis 118:65–73, 1978

24. Mangla PK, Menon MPS: Effect of nasal and oral breathing on exercise-induced asthma. Clin Allergy 11:433–439, 1981

25. Griffin MP, McFadden ER Jr, Ingram RH Jr: Airway cooling in asthmatic and non-asthmatic subjects during nasal and oral breathing. J All Clin Immunol 69:354–359, 1982

26. McFadden ER: Asthma: Airway reactivity and pathogenesis. Semin Respir Med 1:287–296, 1980

27. McNally JR Jr, Enright P, Hirsch JE, et al: The attenuation of exercise-induced bronchocongestion by oropharyngeal anesthesia. Am Rev Respir Dis 119:247–252, 1979

28. Aquilina AT, Hall WJ, Douglas RG, et al: Airway reactivity in subjects with viral upper respiratory tract infections: The effects of exercise and cold air. Am Rev Respir Dis 122:3–10, 1980

29. Enright PL, McNally JF, Souhadra JF: Effect of lidocaine on the ventilatory and airway responses to exercise in asthmatics. Am Rev Respir Dis 122:823–828, 1980

30. Strauss RH, McFadden ER, Ingram RH, et al: Enhancement of exercise-induced asthma by cold air. N Engl J Med 297:734–747, 1977

31. Rodriguez-Martinez F, Mascia AV, Mellins RB: The effect of environmental temperature on airway resistance in the asthmatic child. Pediatr Res 7:627–631, 1973

32.  Fanta CH, Ingram RH, McFadden ED: A reassessment of the effects of oropharyngeal anesthesia in exercise-induced asthma. Am Rev Respir Dis 122:381–386, 1980
33.  Griffin MP, McFadden ER Jr, Ingram RH Jr, et al: Controlled analysis of inhaled lidocaine in exercise-induced asthma. Thorax 37:741–5, 1982.
34.  Acres JC, Kryger: Clinical significance of pulmonary function tests. Chest 80:207–211, 1981
35.  Irwin RS, Rosen MJ, Braman SS: Cough: A comprehensive review. Arch Int Med 137:1186–1191, 1977
36.  Irwin RS, Corrao WM, Pratter MR: Chronic persistent cough in the adult. The spectrum and frequency of causes and successful outcome of specific therapy. Am Rev Respir Dis 123:413–417, 1981
37.  Spector SL, Lotan A, English G, et al: Comparison between transillumination and the roentgenogram in diagnosing paranasal sinus disease. J Allergy Clin Immunol 67:22–26, 1981
38.  Slavin RG, Cannon RE, Friedman WH, et al: Sinusitis and bronchial asthma. J Allergy Clin Immunol 66:250–257, 1980
39.  Mullarkey MF: A clinical approach to rhinitis. Med Clin N Am 65:977–986, 1981
40.  Berg T, Johanson SGO: IgE concentrations in children with atopic diseases. Int Arch Allergy 36:219–232, 1969
41.  Seebohm DM: In Middleton EL, Reed CR, Ellis EF (Eds): Allergy: Principles and Practice, St. Louis, Mosby, CV, 1978, pp 868–876
42.  Zeiger RS, Schatz M: Chronic rhinitis: A practical approach to diagnosis and treatment. Part II: Treatment. Immunol All Pract 4:26–36, 1982
43.  Karlin JM: The use of antihistamines in allergic disease. Pediatr Clin N Am 22:157–162, 1975
44.  Johnstone DE: Study of the role of antigen dosage in the treatment of pollenosis and pollen asthma. Am J Dis Childh 94:1–5, 1957
45.  Jacobs RL, Freedman PM, Boswell RN: Nonallergic rhinitis with eosinophilia (NARES syndrome): Clinical and immunologic presentation. J Allergy Clin Immunol 67:253–262, 1981
46.  Brown BL, Harner SG, Van Dellen RG: Nasal polypectomy in patients with asthma and sensitivity to aspirin. Arch Otolaryngealol 105:413–416, 1979

# 22

ROBERT S. ZEIGER

## Asthma in Childhood

Childhood asthma presents a major therapeutic and sociologic challenge to physician, parent, and child. Approximately 8 million or 12% of all children experience at least one episode of bronchospasm, and about 5% or 3 million suffer from chronic asthma. Seventy percent of affected children have their first attack of asthma before the age of 3 years, and over 50% of adult asthmatics are able to date their asthma to childhood. Asthma is more common in children than in adults, and, for reasons yet to be discovered, males experience considerably more asthma than do females in early childhood, but the incidence equalizes during adolescence.*

### MORBIDITY AND MORTALITY

Childhood asthma accounts for 4.5 million physician visits per year. It is the third most frequent presenting complaint of outpatients visiting the Children's Hospital in Ann Arbor. It results in 58,000 hospitalizations per year (238,000 hospital days) in the United States and has been the most frequent cause of medical admissions to Children's Hospital Medical Center in Boston for many years. Approximately 50 million dollars are spent for medication, 35 million dollars for hospital costs, and more than 100 million dollars for physician fees per year. It causes more than 6 million days of school absence per year. One hundred to two hundred children die each year from status asthmaticus, a figure that could be reduced with more aggressive diagnostic and therapeutic approaches.**

### RISK FACTORS IN CHILDHOOD ASTHMA

The incidence of chronic asthma is 7 times greater in children with a bilateral parental history of allergy (14%) compared to those whose parents have no history of allergy (2%). Parental smoking patterns also affect the occurrence of persistent wheezing

---

*Data from Asthma and the other allergic diseases, NIAID Task Force Report, US Dept HEW, NIH Publ No 79-387, May 1979 Chapter 1.

**Data from Asthma and the other allergic diseases, NIAID Task Force report, US Department, HEW Publ. No 79-387 (May 1979)

**167**

in their children, with a 12% incidence if both parents smoke, a 7% incidence if the mother smokes, and only a 2% incidence if neither smokes.[1] The presence of a decrease in forced expiratory flow in children has recently been shown to correlate with current maternal smoking habits. Lower respiratory tract illnesses such as bronchiolitis and pneumonia are twice as frequent in children with persistent wheeze (28%), and upper respiratory sinus problems are 12 times as common (12%) in the asthmatic child. Bottle-fed babies have a poorer prognosis and a greater incidence of asthma, which is of greater severity, than do infants who are breast fed for more than 2 months.[2] Thirty percent to 78 percent of childhood asthmatics continue to manifest asthma as adults and in 6%–19% of them, the asthma remains moderate to severe.[3] Asthma is more likely to remit in adolescence if it first develops after 3 years of age and before 6–8 years, whereas a poorer prognosis can be expected when the onset of asthma occurs before 2 years or after 10 years of age. The likelihood of remission is less if the child also suffers from atopic dermatitis or allergic rhinitis.[4] Allergic rhinitis and asthma often develop at nearly the same time. For example, only 3% of 528 Denver teenage asthmatics reported rhinitis appearing more than 1 year prior to asthma.[5] These data should dispel the myth that most children will "outgrow" their asthma.

## PATHOPHYSIOLOGY

Asthma produces much the same physiologic alterations in children and in adults, but there are anatomic and physiologic differences in the young child and infant that cause more severe respiratory symptoms that appear more rapidly and lead more frequently to respiratory failure.

### Increased Peripheral Resistance to Airflow

The growth of the infant's airways after birth is enormous. The number of alveoli and airways and the lung surface area increase tenfold from birth to 4–8 years. The diameter of the terminal bronchiole in a 6-month-old infant is 0.1 mm or 20% of its diameter at maturity. Peripheral airways are thus disproportionately narrowed in infancy, and the peripheral resistance to airflow is increased until around age 6. The small airways in infants normally contribute about 70% of the total airflow resistance, in contrast to less than 50% at maturity.[6] As a result, diseases that narrow the small airways will cause a greater increase in pulmonary resistance in infants in comparison to the older child and adult. Although early studies based on examination of a few pathologic bronchial specimens suggested that infants under 1 year of age lacked bronchial smooth muscle, more recent reports demonstrated smooth muscle in the terminal bronchioles of full-term infants.[7] It is still unknown how smooth muscle responds to various stimuli in these infants. Despite some reports that infants as young as 2 months of age can demonstrate a dramatic physiologic improvement with aminophylline[8] or epinephrine, conflicting studies have evolved with respect to the effect of alpha- and beta-adrenergic agents and theophylline on reducing airways resistance in infants under 18 months of age with bronchiolitis or wheezing.[9,10] Mucous glands are more numerous in the major bronchi of young children than in adults and may contribute to increased quantities of mucus and subsequent obstruction.

## Lowered Elastic Recoil Pressure and Early Airway Closure

It has been proposed that infants are susceptible to early airway closure due to a relative lack of lung elastic recoil.[11] The lowered oxygen tension normally occurring in young infants is due to early airway closure. Therefore, a similar degree of inflammation of the airways will cause more profound disturbances in gas exchange during infancy.

## Poorly Developed Collateral Ventilation

There are fewer and smaller interalveolar pores of Kohn and bronchoalveolar (Lambert's) canals and fewer openings between alveolar ducts in the infant lung.[12] Obstructive changes secondary to mucus, edema, inflammatory cells, or spasm are thus more likely to cause atelectasis.

## Thoracic and Diaphragmatic Disadvantages

The horizontal insertion of the infant's diaphragm, in contrast to an oblique insertion in adults, causes the diaphragm to "suck in" the infant's very compliant rib cage rather than to move air into the lungs effectively.[13] The diaphragm has fewer fatique-resistant muscle fibers in the infant than in the adult and thus copes less well with increased workloads.[14]

## CLINICAL MANIFESTATIONS

### Precipitants of Asthma

As in the adult, various stimuli may lead to bronchial hyperreactivity in the asthmatic child. The relative importance of viral infection, inhaled and ingested antigens, and nonspecific stimuli (exercise, irritants, emotion) at different stages during childhood is noted in Table 22-1.

**Table 22-1**
**Precipitants of Asthma: Relative Importance with Respect to Age**

| Precipitant | Age Group | | | |
|---|---|---|---|---|
| | Infancy | Early Childhood | Late Childhood | Adolescence |
| Viral infection | + + + + | + + + | +(+) | +(+) |
| Foods | + + | + | Rare | Rare |
| Indoor inhalants | + | + + + | + + + | + + |
| Pollens | − | + | + + + | + + |
| Exercise or irritants | + | + + | + + + | + + + |

Modified from Pearlman DS, Bierman CW: Asthma (bronchial asthma, reactive airways disorder), in Bierman CW, Pearlman DS (Eds): Allergic Diseases of Infancy, Childhood, and Adolescence. Philadelphia, Saunders, 1980, p 585. With Permission.

## Viral Infections

At least 80% of wheezing before 3 years of age can be attributed to viral infections, most commonly respiratory syncytial virus (RSV). In older children rhinovirus, myxoviruses (parainfluenza, influenza), and mycoplasma appear to be the most frequent infectious agents causing asthma.[15] Asthmatic children have more viral respiratory infections, particularly with rhinovirus, than do their nonasthmatic siblings (5.1 vs 3.8/yr per subject).[16] Viral illnesses were implicated in 9 of 11 children aged 2½–8, who developed severe respiratory failure,[17] and in 64% of children aged 5–15 years requiring corticosteroid treatment.[18] Viruses are recovered more often from sputum than from nose or throat specimens, implying that viral replication occurs more readily in the lower respiratory tract.[18] Bacterial infections seldom trigger acute asthma, but they may complicate an existing viral illness.

Recent studies have led to a better understanding of the mechanism of virus-induced wheezing. For several weeks after uncomplicated viral respiratory infections, normal subjects show increased smooth-muscle reactivity and a decreased cough threshold when challenged with bronchoconstrictor aerosols,[19] cold air, or exercise.[20] It has been suggested that viral infection damages the bronchial epithelium and thus sensitizes the exposed rapidly adapting sensory receptors since these abnormal responses are abolished by previous treatment with atropine. More recently, RSV specific IgE was found in nasopharyngeal secretions in about 70% of 60 infants with wheezing during RSV infection and in only 5% of infants who did not wheeze. Histamine was detectable significantly more often and in greater concentration in nasopharyngeal secretions from wheezing than nonwheezing infants. Moreover, peak RSV-IgE titers and histamine concentration appeared to correlate significantly with the extent of hypoxia.[21] The capability of viruses to stimulate the formation of specific viral IgE which binds to and persists on respiratory tissue and can subsequently trigger specific histamine release identifies a true IgE mechanism by which infection with viruses such as RSV may cause wheezing.

Acute bronchiolitis is an obstructive inflammation of the bronchioli and small bronchi, caused mainly by RSV. It is most common in infants 2–6 months of age, frequently is the initial manifestation of bronchospasm, and often is indistinguishable from asthma. Although bronchiolitis occurs in only a small percentage of infants during RSV epidemics, recurrent wheezing occurs in 30%–50% of those infants who have been hospitalized.[22] Elevated serum IgE levels and atopic family history appear to serve as a reliable predictor of subsequent wheezing in infants with bronchiolitis, although a recent study disagrees with these earlier observations.[23] Acute viral bronchiolitis may be recurrent, but when there are repeated episodes of "bronchiolitis" in infancy, asthma should be suspected. There was clinical evidence of bronchiolitis in 38% of primary RSV viral infections, but the severity of the illness tended to diminish with each reinfection.[24] There were persistent abnormalities of lung function [abnormal $PaO_2$, residual volume/total lung capacity (RV/TLC), and volume of isoflow] in the majority of symptom-free nonasthmatic children 10 years after severe bronchiolitis in infancy requiring hospitalization. These changes indicate residual lesions in the parenchyma or the airways following severe bronchiolitis.[25]

## Croup

Acute laryngotracheobronchitis (croup) is a common condition caused by acute adductor spasm of the vocal cords that leads to inspiratory stridor, a barking or brassy cough, hoarseness, and occasionally respiratory distress due to laryngeal obstruction.

Spirometric measurements in children hospitalized with croup in infancy 8.5 years previously were significantly different from those of normal children. Moreover, 35% of these children who had had croup had abnormal bronchial hyperreactivity as determined by methacholine challenge testing.[26] Children with recurrent croup have an increased incidence of airway hyperreactivity and reduced expiratory flow rates and are significantly more likely to develop allergies or asthma.[27] These findings suggest that recurrent croup, like asthma, should be considered a manifestation of hyperreactive airways.[28]

### Allergens

The role of allergens in asthma is discussed in Chapters 7 and 18, but several points are of special importance in children. The allergens triggering asthma in infancy appear to be foodstuffs, particularly milk and egg proteins, as demonstrated by skin testing and double-blind challenges. The offending foods should be avoided during infancy. Foods become less important as causative agents in older children, and often there is spontaneous remission of the food allergy by age 3. Allergies to inhaled substances have been demonstrated within the first year of life, but generally sensitization to indoor inhalants (mold, dust, and danders) occurs in early childhood and to outdoor inhalants (pollen) in later childhood. There had often been an acute viral illness during the month preceding allergic sensitization in allergy-prone infants. Specific IgE antibodies can be demonstrated in 75%–90% of childhood asthmatics, with a higher incidence in the more severely affected, suggesting that allergies have an important role in triggering asthma.

### Nonspecific Triggers

Exercise has been shown to provoke bronchospasm in 63% of asthmatic children and in 41% of atopic children who have no history of asthma.[29] Exercise-induced asthma is thus very frequent in allergic children and adolescents, but spirometry following an exercise challenge may be required before the diagnosis can be confirmed. Exercise-induced asthma is most common in later childhood and adolescence probably because of increased activities during this period of life. Swimming is the least asthmagenic exercise, probably because the inhalation of warm, moist air is less likely to trigger bronchospasm than the cold, dry air inhaled during running and bicycling.[30]

Irritants such as cigarette smoke, fumes, air pollutants, and chemicals are similarly noxious to children with asthma. Since children are usually the passive recipients of these irritants, it is the responsibility of their parents or guardians to protect them. Aspirin idiosyncracy (asthma, nasal polyps, and aspirin sensitivity) has been demonstrated in older children and adolescents but is less frequent than in adults. However, aspirin ingestion may decrease forced expiratory flow in up to 30% of children and adolescents with severe asthma;[31] thus aspirin-containing products and nonsteroidal anti-inflammatory agents should be avoided unless there is good medical reason for their use. Tartrazine sensitivity is as uncommon in children as in adults. Although psychological factors may influence the course of asthma in certain children, the effects of severe asthma on the emotional development of children and their relationships with their families are of far greater importance.

### Gastroesophageal Reflux

Gastroesophageal reflux, or distal esophageal dysfunction causing frequent return of stomach contents into the esophagus, occurs in about 1 in every 500 infants.[32] Its incidence increases to between 30%–70% in patients with recurrent pneumonia or chronic asthma.[33]

Gastroesophageal reflux may act as a nonspecific trigger in some children. The diagnosis depends on clinical awareness supported by positive results in more than one of the following procedures: acid reflux test, esophageal manometry, video esophagram with upper gastrointestinal (GI) series, esophagoscopy, and esophageal biopsy. These tests should be performed after discontinuation of oral bronchodilators, including theophylline and beta-adrenergic agents, if possible, because both of these medications reduce lower esophageal sphincter pressure. Medical measures to control reflux include utilizing the elevated prone positioning $(30°)$[32] and thickened feedings in the infant, and oral antacids, and $H_2$-receptor antagonists in older children. Cholinergic agents such as oral Urecholine (Merck Sharp & Dohme, Westpoint, PA) may be considered to prevent GER; however, in a small percentage of asthmatics, cholinergics may exacerbate asthma. Surgical antireflux therapy (fundoplication) has been successful in patients with severe pulmonary disorders and proven esophagitis who have not responded to medical treatment.[33]

## Clinical Presentations

Many clinical patterns, frequently varying with age, are seen in childhood asthma. Wheezing with accompanying coarse adventitious sounds on auscultation, rib retraction, and tachypnea are the characteristic signs of asthma in infancy. Not infrequently, the infant appears unperturbed by these symptoms, but they should be treated since respiratory reserve in infants is low and respiratory failure often develops rapidly. Nighttime coughing also occurs in the infant asthmatic but is usually associated with rib retraction and wheezing.[15]

In the older child and the adolescent, chronic cough may be the only manifestation of airway hyperreactivity.[34] Many of these patients have normal resting spirometric measurements that are unchanged after isoproterenol. Exercise challenge sometimes produces spirometric changes in these "cough patients" similar to those observed in other asthmatics. Hannaway and Hopper[35] studied 32 patients referred for evaluation of cough and found that they improved with theophylline. Shapiro et al.[36] found increased sensitivity to methacholine in 66% of 160 young subjects with symptoms suggestive of lower respiratory problems but normal spirometry. Since it is impracticable to treat all patients with chronic cough, these authors suggest that a methacholine bronchial challenge will identify the patients who may benefit from bronchodilator treatment.

McNicol and Williams[37] studied prospectively a randomly selected group of over 300 children with wheezing. Factors associated with more severe disease, especially in males, were more frequent attacks that appeared early in life, persistent rhonchi, chest deformities, pulmonary hyperinflation, and growth retardation. Hauspie et al.[38] studied 531 institutionalized asthmatic boys aged 2–20 years of age. Only 3.5% were treated with long-term corticosteroids, none within 3.5 years of the study. They noted that growth in height showed no retardation until childhood, a more pronounced delay at adolescence, and a catch-up growth toward adulthood. Bone age and pubic hair development were also retarded. It is not known whether these maturational delays are secondary to the asthma or are intrinsic abnormalities due to a similar basic defect. Since these patterns of more severe disease emerge by 7 years and are certainly established by 10 years, they must be recognized early so that the patient can be treated aggressively. As a testimony to this urgency, recent studies have identified a group of asthmatic children with reactive airways who have an irreversible obstructive component to their disease despite vigorous bronchodilation and high-dose corticosteroid treatment.[39]

During acute asthma in children supraclavicular indrawing and sternocleidomastoid contraction were more indicative of severe spirometric abnormalities than were signs of subjective dyspnea, wheezing, prolonged expiration or ausculatory rhonchi. When combined with other findings of proven value, such as pulsus paradoxus and arterial blood gases, these physical signs indicate the need for aggressive therapy for prevention of respiratory failure.[40]

More than 20% of the children hospitalized with acute asthma have an abnormal chest radiograph. The most frequent abnormalities are perihilar infiltrates and atelectasis, especially of the right middle lobe. These findings were most common in the younger children. Pneumomediastinum was the third most common abnormality in older children and adolescents, but it was not seen in infants.[41]

## DIFFERENTIAL DIAGNOSIS

Although most episodes of wheezing in childhood are due to asthma, other less common causes of wheezing are listed in Table 22-2. Their relative frequency at differing stages of childhood is noted in Table 22-3. Upper and lower respiratory tract infections,

**Table 22-2**
**Differential Diagnosis of Obstructive Respiratory Disorders in Children**

| Category | Specific Entity |
| --- | --- |
| Upper Respiratory | |
|   Congenital | Tracheal stenosis, larynogotracheomalacia, vascular ring, vocal cord paresis |
|   Aspiration | Foreign body*, vomitus, reflux |
|   Infection | Laryngotracheobronchitis*, epiglottitis*, laryngitis, peritonsillar abscess, nasopharyngitis-sinusitis* |
|   Tumor | Papilloma, hemangioma, lymphangioma, teratoma, severe tonsillar and adenoidal hypertrophy, polyps |
|   Miscellaneous | Irritative (aspiration, drowning, intubation), laryngospasm, allergic angioedema, hereditary angioneurotic edema, tetany, noxious gas inhalation, psychogenic |
| Lower Respiratory | |
|   Congenital | Bronchostenosis, bronchomalacia, lobar emphysema, aberrant vessels, cystic fibrosis, immune deficiency |
|   Aspiration | Foreign body*, tracheoesophageal fistula, Riley-Day syndrome, hiatus hernia, drowning, vomitus, esophageal reflux |
|   Infection | Bronchiolitis*, pneumonia*, pertussis, TB, bronchiectasis |
|   Tumors | Bronchogenic cyst, teratoma, atrial myxoma, carcinoid |
|   Immunologic | Asthma*, allergic bronchopulmonary aspergillosis, hypersensitivity pneumonitis |
|   Miscellaneous | Right middle-lobe syndrome*, cardiac failure, toxic gaseous inhalation, pneumothorax, pulmonary embolism, hyperventilation (acute salicylism, acidosis, psychogenic) |

*More frequently seen entities
Modified from Simons FER: Asthma in children. Semin Respir Med 1:*149* 1979. With permission.

**Table 22-3**
**Relative Frequency of Occurrence or Age of Diagnosis of Common Childhood Disorders**
**Requiring Differentiation from Asthma**

| Disorder | Infancy | Childhood | Adolescence |
|---|---|---|---|
| Laryngotracheobronchomalacia | + + | ± | − |
| Bronchiolitis | + + + | + + | − |
| Chronic viral/chlamydial infection | + + + | + + | − |
| Congenital abnormalities | + + + | + | − |
| Aspiration (chalasia) | + + + | + | − |
| Cystic fibrosis | + + + | + | − |
| Pertussis syndrome | + + + | + | ± |
| Chronic bacterial nasopharyngitis sinusitis | + + + | + + | + |
| Croup | + + | + | ± |
| Epiglottitis | + + | + + | ± |
| Foreign body | + | + + | ± |
| Hyperventilation syndrome | − | + | + + + |
| Mitral valve prolapse | − | − | + |

Modified from Pearlman DS, Bierman CW: Asthma (bronchial asthma, reactive airways disorder), in Bierman CW, Pearlman DS (Eds): Allergic Diseases of Infancy, Childhood, and Adolescence. Philadelphia, Saunders, 1980, p 590. With permission.

which may mimic asthma, are common in infancy and early childhood. Chronic chlamydial penumonia in infancy has been recognized more often since the late 1970s and is characterized by a dry hacking cough, chronic pulmonary infiltrates, elevated immunoglobulins in the serum, and an afebrile nontoxic course that responds to combined erythromycin and sulfisoxazole.[42]

A raucous bronchial cough occurs characteristically with chronic nasopharnygitis or sinusitis since secretions are less frequently coughed up and expelled in infants and young children. A proportion of patients with cystic fibrosis, perhaps 10%, have no GI abnormalities or chronic pulmonary infections and are seen by the allergist with an illness indistinguishable from typical asthma. Congenital malformation (tracheal webs, vascular rings, etc.) should be suspected when there are abnormal auscultatory sounds during both inspiration and expiration in a patient who is not acutely ill. Acute inspiratory and expiratory stridor may be seen with foreign bodies, in severe Stage IV asthma, and when croup occurs in an asthmatic.

## KEY DIAGNOSTIC TESTS

Diagnostic procedures particularly helpful in differentiating the various causes of persistent wheezing in childhood are noted in Table 22-4. Most of them are also used in adults. Skin testing techniques, spirometry, bronchial challenge, and cytologic examination of secretions are discussed in earlier chapters. Although puncture skin testing in

Table 22-4
**Diagnostic Procedures Frequently Revealing in Children with Persistent Wheezing**

| Procedure | Disorder |
|---|---|
| Asthma, croup, laryngomalacia | Spirometry ± exercise |
| Allergic vs infectious | Nasal-sputum cytology |
| Atopy | Allergen skin tests |
| Food allergy | Food avoidance trial |
| Parenchymal lung or cardiac disease | Chest x-ray |
| Foreign body | Inspiratory-expiratory chest x-ray |
| Sinusitis | Water's sinus x-ray |
| TE* fistula, vascular ring, aspiration, chalasia, gastroesophageal reflux | Barium swallow |
| Gastroesophageal Reflux | Tuttle test |
| Pulmonary Hemosiderosis | Hemosiderin macrophages and milk precipitins |
| Cystic Fibrosis | Sweat test—ionotophoresis |
| Immune Deficiency | Quantitative Immunoglobulins and delayed hypersensitivity tests |

*Tracheoesophageal.

infants has been discouraged, appropriately performed testing with selected foods (milk, egg, wheat, corn, soy, and peanut) and environmental (alternaria, hormodendrum, mite, dander, and grass) allergens by use of a Multitest (Lincoln) puncture device is simple and helps to predict later atopic manifestations. We have found about an 80% correlation between positive multitest puncture tests and radioallergosorbent (RAST) testing in infants less than 1 year of age. More than 50% of children over age 3 with positive puncture tests to food allergens and a history of food-induced symptoms show an immediate reaction to food challenge, whereas negative food puncture tests are typically accompanied by negative double-blind food challenges. Gastrointestinal symptoms generally precede or accompany food-induced respiratory symptoms.[43]

Examination of nasal cytology using a Rhinoprobe (Rhinotechnics, San Diego, CA) and the sputum is useful if it shows eosinophils, neutrophils with or without bacteria inclusions, or basophilic cell infiltration.[43a] The presence of mast cells could help to predict a response to therapeutic measures, especially cromolyn.

## TREATMENT

### General Measures

A number of general principles, which are often glossed over by the physician, are of great importance in any therapeutic program.

Successful therapy of the asthmatic child must include the patient's parents. Unless both the parents and the child understand and agree to the treatment, it is doomed to failure. Educational tools such as video recordings, booklets, and lecture sessions can be used to instruct them about asthma. Daily symptom and medication diaries provide objective evidence of the success or failure of the regimen, improve compliance, and reduce emergency room visits and hospitalizations.

Even if provoking factors can be avoided, most asthmatic children will require at least intermittent use of medications. A beta-2 agonist may suffice, but if the asthma is chronic, combinations of cromolyn, theophylline, and beta-2 agonists are often needed.

Only a few childhood asthmatics will require chronic corticosteroids, and a few patients may ultimately be placed on immunotherapy. Details of using these agents follow.

An effective approach for the more recalcitrant patient is outlined in Table 22-5. Childhood asthmatics must be assured and then convinced by successful treatment that the illness does not make them handicapped people. They must learn enough about the disease and assume enough responsibility for their care that self-sufficiency can be achieved during adolescence. Noncompliance can be a serious problem in children, but it can be managed by behavioral modification with reward reinforcement. Recording of daily peakflows at home with an inexpensive, portable peakflow whistle or similar device can often aid in recognizing worsening asthma. The adolescent, on the other hand, must be convinced of the importance of adhering to a medical regimen. Team swimming for 1–2 hours at least 5 days each week has been shown to reduce asthma symptoms and

**Table 22-5**
**Treatment of Recalcitrant Childhood Asthma**

| Clues | Approach |
|---|---|
| Disease Characteristics | |
| Physical stigmata | Confirm diagnosis |
| Relative fixed airway obstruction | Maximize treatment |
| Partial response to steroids | Elective hospitalization |
| Additional complicating illnesses | Rule out thyroid, cystic fibrosis etc. |
| Failure of previous medical care | Contact physician |
| Failure of immunotherapy | Evaluate regimen |
| | |
| Family Dynamics | |
| Passive or neglectful mother | Confrontation (need child advocate) |
| Maternal–Paternal conflict | Invite dual involvement |
| Parental–Child conflict | Counseling |
| Single parent | Support services |
| Smoking parent | Discontinue |
| | |
| Patient Involvement | |
| Denial (low panic fear) | Confrontation |
| Ignorance | Education |
| Noncompliance | Theophylline levels, peak flow at home |
| High panic fear | Reassurance |
| Unrealistic expectations | Recognize own limitations |
| Inactive or inappropriate physical activity | Encourage swimming regularly |

medication requirements, often with improvement in pulmonary function.[30] Avoidance of provoking factors (parental and patient smoking, irritants, and allergens) may be especially rewarding in children. Every effort should be made to control the environment, and a home visit by a trained environmental nurse may be warranted. Spirometry is no less important in children than in adults for following the success of the treatment program. Children as young as 4 years of age can adequately perform the forced expiratory maneuver, and normal spirometric values are available for young children.

## Specific Therapy

The same medications are used to treat children and adults with asthma but there are differences in the dosage, in the frequency of side effects, and in the ages at which the various bronchodilators work best (Table 22-6).

### *Theophyllines (Table 22-7)*

The dosage of theophylline in the pediatric asthmatic must be carefully adjusted because of the great individual and age-related variations in the clearance rate. Dosage guidelines for intravenous (IV) and oral routes are noted in Table 22-7. In the child less than 18 months of age, one must prove that the drug is effective before committing the child to maintenance therapy. A recent retrospective study of hospitalized children under 18 months of age was unable to reveal any beneficial effect of theophylline on the resolution of acute bronchiolitis.[44] It is difficult to distinguish bronchiolitis from acute asthma in the individual patient, and because some asthmatics less than 18 months of age improve with theophylline,[8] it is probably best to give the drug a trial.

Several of the available theophylline preparations are listed in Chapter 8. Aminophylline U.S.P. (21 mg/ml theophylline equivalent) and most recently, predissolved 100% theophylline (Travenol Laboratories Deerfield, IL) are the only theophylline formulations available for IV use. Theophylline suppositories are unpredictably absorbed, but the rectal solution of aminophylline (51 mg/ml theophylline content; Somophylline rectal Solution, Fisons Corporation, Bedford, MA) provides a convenient, rapid, and consistent route for theophylline administration in a frightened young child with relatively inaccessible veins. Peak theophylline concentrations are obtained within 1–2 hours after the rectal solution is given.

**Table 22-6**
**Special Problems with Pharmacologic Agents Inherent in Childhood Asthma**

Relatively poorer bronchodilator response in infants

Relatively frequent medication intolerance in infancy and early childhood.
  Nightmares and/or sleep walking (theophyllines, beta-adrenergics)

  Behavioral disturbances (theophyllines, beta-adrenergics)

  Poorer retention during learning (?)

  Growth retardation (corticosteroids)

Difficulty of inhaler use

Parent–child conflict over compliance

**Table 22-7**
**Pharmacologic Agents and Dosages in Childhood Asthma**

| Agent | Parenteral | Oral | Aerosol Inhalation |
|---|---|---|---|
| | | Administration (Route) | |
| **Beta-Adrenergic** | | | |
| Epinephrine | Subcutaneous: 1 mg/ml (1:1000) solution: 0.01 ml/kg q15–q20 min × 3 prn (max. 0.4 ml) | No | Not indicated |
| Susphrine | Subcutaneous: 5 mg/ml (1:200) solution: 0.005 ml/kg ≥q4–q6 h (max. 0.15 ml) 20% rapid and 80% sustained release | No | Not indicated |
| Isoproterenol* | Intravenous: 0.2 mg/ml (0.02%) solution | No | 5 mg/ml (0.5%) solution use 0.01 ml/kg to a maximum of 0.5 ml diluted with 1.5-ml saline q2–6 h |
| | Continuous pump infusion: 0.1 $\mu g/(kg\ min^{-1})$ initial dose, increase by 0.1 $\mu g/kg/min$ at intervals of 15 min until $PaCO_2$ falls, P > 200, diastolic BP < 40 mm Hg, or 0.8 $\mu g/(kg\ min^{-1})$ | | |
| Isoetharine* | Not available | No | 10 mg/ml (1%) solution dosage same as for isoproterenol |
| Metaproterenol* | Subcutaneous: 0.5 mg/ml (0.05%) solution‡ 0.04 ml/kg q 30 min × 3 prn | 10 mg/5 ml syrup or 10 mg tablet, 0.3–0.5 mg/kg per dose q6–8 h | 50 mg/ml (5%) solution use 0.005–0.010 ml/kg to a maximum of 0.3 ml, diluted with 1.5 ml saline and given 4–6 times daily† |

| | | | |
|---|---|---|---|
| Terbutaline | Subcutaneous: 1.0 mg/ml (0.1%) solution 0.01 ml/kg q30 min × 3 prn (max. 0.4 ml) | 0.3 mg/ml syrup‡ or 2.5 mg tablet, 0.1–0.15 mg/kg per dose q6–8 h | 10 mg/ml (1%) solution use 0.03 ml/kg to a maximum of 1 ml, diluted as above and given 4–6 times daily† |
| Albuterol* (Salbutamol) | Intravenous: 1 mg/ml (0.1%) solution‡<br><br>Bolus: 10 $\mu$g/kg diluted and given over 10 min<br><br>Continuous pump infusion: 0.2 $\mu$g/(kg min$^{-1}$) increasing by 0.1 $\mu$g/(kg min$^{-1}$) q15 min to a maximum of 2 $\mu$g/(kg min$^{-1}$) | 2 mg/5 ml syrup‡ or 2 mg tablet, 0.1–0.15 mg/kg per dose q6–8 h | 5 mg/ml (0.5%) solution‡ use 0.03 ml/kg to a maximum of 1 ml, diluted as above 4–6 times daily† |
| Theophylline | Intravenous: (aminophylline U.S.P., 25 mg aminophylline/ml)<br><br>Loading dose: 6–7.5 mg/kg over 20–30 min (if no prior theophylline for 24 hours) or 1 mg/kg for each 2 $\mu$g/ml increase desired in previous serum theophylline concentration<br><br>Continuous infusion: (after loading dose for target concentration of theophylline of 10 $\mu$g/ml), determine level at 6 and 18 h | Anhydrous theophylline preparation preferred, starting dosage (>1 yr): 16 mg/kg or 400 mg daily (whichever is less)<br><br>Increase by 25% increments q3 days if tolerated<br>Sustained-release products preferred for chronic therapy<br><br>Maximum oral doses before theophylline level required | No |

Table 22-7
(Continued)

| Agent | Administration (Route) | | |
|---|---|---|---|
| | Parenteral | Oral | Aerosol Inhalation |
| Theophylline (continued) | Continuous infusion | Maximum oral doses before theophylline level required | |
| | Aminophylline (mg/(kg h$^{-1}$)) | Age / Dose (mg/kg Daily) | |
| | Age | Age / Dose | |
| | Neonate — 0.16 | <1 yr — $8 + 0.3$ times age in weeks | |
| | Infants 2–6 mos — 0.50 | 1–9 — 24 | |
| | Infants 6–11 mos — 0.80 | 9–12 — 20 | |
| | Children 1–9 yr — 1.0 | 12–16 — 18 | |
| | Children >9 years and otherwise healthly adults who smoke — 0.75 | >16 — 13 or 900 mg/day (whichever is less) | |
| | Otherwise healthy nonsmoking adults — 0.50 | | |
| | Cardiac decompensation and liver dysfunction — 0.25 | | |
| Cromolyn sodium | No | No | 10 mg/ml (1%) solution 2 ml 4 times daily |
| Anticholinergic Atropine | Not studied | 0.02 mg/kg per dose q6–8 h | 0.03–0.05 mg/kg per dose dissolve required number of atropine tablets in 2.0 ml saline or use atropine solution from injectable vials |
| Ipratropium bromide‡ | No | No | 250 μg nebulized 4 times daily, or 20–40 μg q6 h in metered dose inhaler‡ |

| Corticosteroid | Intravenous | | |
|---|---|---|---|
| Hydrocortisone succinate (Solucortef) | Loading dose: 5–7 mg/kg diluted in saline over 15 min<br>Maintenance: 4 mg/kg q4 h | No | No |
| Methylprednisolone succinate (Solumedrol) | Loading dose: 1 mg/kg diluted in saline over 15 min<br>Maintenance: 0.8 mg/kg q4 h | No | No |
| Prednisone (prednisolone, methyl prednisolone) | No | 2 mg/kg Daily to start; usually bid; Taper off entirely or to minimally effective alternate-day dosage; Long-term daily dosage unacceptable | No |
| Flunisolide | No | No | 250 µg/ml solution§ Ages <6: Safety not yet established<br>Ages 6–14 yr: 500 µg 2–4 times daily |
| Beclomethasone dipropionate | No | No | Available only as a freon-propelled dose inhaler providing 42 µg per metered dose, 50–100 µg, 2–4 times daily; Dose ≤13 µg/kg per 24 h |

*Available as freon-propelled metered-dose inhaler for older children (see Chapter 9).

†May administer for 5–10 minutes every half hour ×4, every hour ×4, then every 2 hours as indicated by patient's condition, discontinuing if pulse ≥200/minute (see text).

‡Unavailable in United States at this time.

§Available as Nasalide (Syntex Laboratories Inc., Palo Alto, CA) solution for intranasal use.

Although liquid preparations are convenient for the young child, they have several disadvantages, including the high alcohol content (to increase palatability and solubility); high dye, sugar, and preservative content; and the short duration of action. Liquid theophylline preparations containing no alcohol, sugar, or dyes, include Slo-phyllin 80 syrup (anhydrous theophylline solution, 5.3 mg/ml [William H. Rorer, Inc., Fort Washington, PA]) and Elixicon (Berlex Laboratories, Wayne, NJ) suspension (20 mg/ml). The more concentrated liquid theophyllines are less palatable, and there is more risk of toxicity from small errors in dosage. A chewable tablet, Theophyl (Knoll Pharmaceutical Company, Whippany, NJ) (100 mg of theophylline) has been introduced to overcome some of the disadvantages of liquids, but the child may refuse it because of its bitter taste.

For chronic therapy, sustained-release preparations help to overcome the rapid theophylline clearance in childhood, giving more stable blood levels. The less frequent dosing improves compliance. Almost all children above age 4 can be taught to swallow tablets and capsules, but those who cannot can be given the beads from certain sustained-release formulations (Slo-bid [Rorer], Somophyllin-CRT [Fisons Corporation, Bedford, MA] or Theodur Sprinkle [Key Pharmaceuticals Inc. Miami, FL]) sprinkled on a spoonful of palatable soft food washed down with fluid. The sustained release properties will be maintained as long as the beads are not chewed.[45]

The low therapeutic index of theophylline is particularly evident in children. The therapeutically desirable blood theophylline levels of 10–20 $\mu$g/ml may be associated with unacceptable side effects. A recent double-blind study noted that the addition of submaximal doses (mean serum level 8 $\mu$g/ml) of sustained-release theophylline to previous treatment with a beta-2 agonist gave further relief of asthmatic symptoms and improved morning spirometry without appreciable side effects. As such, lower serum levels of theophylline (<10 $\mu$g/ml) may be a safe compromise between efficacy and toxicity in children with asthma. In addition to the typical GI effects, sleep disturbances (insomnia, sleep walking, and nightmares), hyperactivity (irritability and behavioral problems), and impaired school performance are not uncommon side effects of theophylline in children. Over 95% of cases of theophylline intoxication in the pediatric age group were due to overdosing with rectal suppositories in young children (mean age 30 months) occasionally accidental but most often iatrogenic.[46] Rectal solutions of theophylline should *not* be used at home, and the concentrated liquid preparation, if employed at all, must be administered to young children with extreme caution. There is no real evidence that young children are any more sensitive to theophylline than are older children, but enormous dosage errors are possible in the very young because of low body weight. In children, though not in adults, theophylline toxicity is invariably manifest by GI symptoms before seizures develop. Hematemesis can occur in infants, although it is uncommon in adults.

When theophylline is used to treat a pregnant asthmatic, it may affect her child. Placental transfer of theophylline is complete,[47] and since the mean theophylline half-life in 1-day-old neonates is 26 ± 0.7 hours (6 times longer than in the 1-year-old), there is a real risk of fetal side effects from placentally passed theophylline. Infants born to mothers with maternal concentrations of theophylline greater than 12 $\mu$g/ml should be observed for the pharmacologic actions of theophylline. The transfer of theophylline through the breast is about 70%. Breast-fed infants have exhibited irritability and fretful sleeping on days their mothers have taken theophylline, proving that enough of the drug contaminates the breast milk to provide a pharmacologic dose to the nursing infant.

### Beta-Adrenergic Agents (Table 22-7)

Most children under 18 months of age with wheezing do not appear to respond as well to adrenergic bronchodilators. Nebulized albuterol, adrenaline, and phenylephrine failed to reduce total respiratory resistance in all infants less than 18 months of age, whereas albuterol did cause more than a 20% reduction in resistance in 18 of 20 children over 20 months of age.[9] More recently, using a whole-body plethysmograph, 5 of 8 infants less than 1 year of age showed a definite improvement in specific airway conductance studied during an acute episode of wheezing after inhaled albuterol.[10] However, in 32 infants (aged 1 to 12 months) hospitalized with acute wheezing, albuterol alone appeared no better than a placebo in ameliorating the episode. On the other hand, intramuscularly administered dexamethasone (0.3 mg/kg on admission and then 0.1 mg/kg q 8 h) when added to albuterol therapy produced a potentiating effect on the beta-adrenergic responsiveness of these infants resulting in a markedly improved clinical course. Dexamthasone by itself exerted no such beneficial response.[10] Such studies suggest a relative hyporesponsiveness to beta-agonists in these infants asthmatics. There are undoubtedly children between 12 and 18 months of age who do benefit from and deserve a trial of these beta-2 stimulant drugs, but these drugs are probably less effective in the first year of life, and may require added corticosteroids for optimal effectiveness.

Oral administration of beta-two agonists is effective in childhood. Albuterol (2 mg thrice daily in children under 40 pounds and 4 mg thrice daily in those greater than 40 pounds) was found in a double-blind study in 14 asthmatic children (3–6 years of age) to reduce symptom scores and medication use and to improve spirometry while producing mild increases in heart rate, tremor, and irritability.[48] Metaproterenol in children of all ages and terbutaline[49] in children over 6 years have also been shown in double-blind studies to be effective, and there was no evidence of clinically significant tolerance after long-term administration.[50] Metaproterenol improved pulmonary function without increased side effects when added to moderate doses of theophylline in asthmatic children.[51] Orally administered beta agonists can cause behavioral problems at school and home, as well as tremor, headache, anxiety, and palpitations. These side effects can often be reduced if the medication is given by inhalation.

The newer selective beta-two agonists such as terbutaline and albuterol have similar pharmacologic properties and have rather high therapeutic indices when used by inhalation in children. Arrhythmias and sudden death have not been reported in children with these newer aerosolized beta-two agonists. Topical aerosols of these agents can be generated by a compressor-powered nebulizer (Pulmo-Aide [DeVilbiss] or Maxi-Myst [Mead Johnson Pharmaceutical Division, Evansville, IL] systems). Aerosol nebulization is effective for both the acutely asthmatic outpatient and for the home management of asthma in children too young to master the use of a metered-dose inhaler. The effect is rapid (within minutes) and may last for 4–6 hours. Tremor and irritability may occur with aerosolized beta-two agonists but are much less frequent and severe than after oral administration.

Garra et al.[52] administered by aerosolization a 0.5% metaproterenol solution for 5 minutes every half hour for 2 hours, hourly for 4 hours, and then every 2 hours as needed for the next 18 hours to 15 childhood asthmatics hospitalized for status asthmaticus. Isoproterenol (0.05% solution) was administered in the same manner for comparison in this double-blind study. The mean maximum pulse rate after metaproterenol treatment was 174 beats per minute. Treatment did not need to be stopped in any of the patients because of a heart rate exceeding 200 beats per minute. The metaproterenol aerosol treatment was safer and produced a more sustained improvement in pulmonary function than did isoproterenol. The safety of such frequent administration of metaproterenol should stimulate a more aggressive use of beta-two agents by nebulization during acute status asthmaticus. Schwartz et al.[53] examined the efficacy of subcutaneous epinephrine and terbutaline or inhaled isoetharine in the treatment of acute asthma in 169 patients in a children's emergency room. Inhaled beta-adrenergic agents were found to be as effective as subcutaneous epinephrine or terbutaline and thus should be considered a safer alternative to the standard injected drugs. The more selective beta-two agonists, metaproterenol, terbutaline, and albuterol, probably would offer an even greater therapeutic index.

### Cromolyn Sodium (Cromolyn) (Table 22-7)

Cromolyn, delivered as powder by a Spinhaler®, has been the preferred drug for prophylaxis of chronic childhood asthma in Great Britain for over a decade. It has been less accepted in the United States, although studies in both countries demonstrate a similar success rate (52%–89% range).[54] More recently several double-blind studies (reported in 1980) have shown that nebulized 1% cromolyn solution (20 mg in 2 ml of water) is an effective form of therapy for childhood asthmatics aged 1 to 7 years who previously were denied cromolyn because of technical restraints. Several double-blind studies have demonstrated that nebulizer cromolyn significantly prevented or inhibited both allergen and exercise-triggered asthma to a degree similar to powdered cromolyn delivered by spinhaler in older children (mean age 12). Exercise induced wheezing in 13/14 preschool childhood asthmatics (mean age 4 years) was abated also by nebulizer cromolyn.[55] Nebulizer cromolyn 1% solution (Intal Nebulizer Solution [Fisons]) is now available in the United States. The solution may be delivered by face mask (or a mouthpiece in older children) with a compressor-powered nebulizer.

Nebulizer cromolyn was significantly better than a placebo at controlling cough and wheezing, at increasing symptom-free days, at improving activity and at improving pulmonary function in 62 young childhood asthmatics.[55a,b] In addition, nebulizer cromolyn was found to be at least as effective as theophylline in controlling asthmatic symptoms while reducing adverse effects in infants and young children (1–6 year olds).[55c] The effectiveness of long-term chronic administration of nebulizer cromolyn in controlling asthma in 16 young children (2–7 year olds) with chronic mixed asthma was documented by a reduced frequency of emergency visits ($p < 0.01$), corticosteroid courses, and hospitalizations during the same six month interval (August through February) compared to prior to such treatment.[55d] The safety of nebulizer cromolyn in these young childhood asthmatics was established by infrequent minor side effects (hyperventilation, inconvenience of frequency of administration) and absence of any significant alteration in hematologic, liver, or renal function.[55a-d] Though nebulizer cromolyn should ideally be administered 4 times daily for optimal therapy, many children can be maintained on twice or three times daily treatments. In addition to the infant and young child, nebulizer cromolyn has proven beneficial to the older child who has not benefited from spinhaler cromolyn either due to inadequate technique or irritative cough from the powder. Given the not infrequent adverse effects secondary from theophylline and oral beta-adrenergic agents in infants and young children, judicious and early intervention with nebulizer cromolyn therapy appears particularly warranted. Bronchodilators (beta-adrenergic and/or anticholinergic agents) can be conveniently nebulized when cough or wheezing occur. It appears unnecessary to discontinue nebulizer cromolyn at these times since no additional irritation appears with its usage. Its potential to inhibit further mast cell release can therefore be maintained during these exacerbations, though studies are necessary to determine the efficacy of this suggestion. Future studies are needed to determine the benefit of nebulizer cromolyn for infectious asthma and in infants less than age one. Cromolyn overall offers the advantages of safety and a low incidence of side effects in comparison to theophylline and the oral beta-adrenergics.

### Anticholinergic Agents (Table 22-7)

Atropine has been used in asthmatic children, both orally and by inhalation, in an attempt to block the vagally mediated component of irritant-induced bronchospasm. Single-dose usage of nebulized atropine sulfate (0.025 to 0.05 mg/kg) has been an effective bronchodilator that acts less rapidly than isoetharine, but its action is better sustained 3 hours after administration.[56] However, chronic use of nebulized atropine for 3 months in a lower dose of 0.02 mg/kg three times daily was not effective. The lower maintenance dose was selected because larger amounts caused blurred vision and dry mouth in many patients. Oral atropine in the same dose (0.02 mg/kg tid) significantly improved spirometric measurements in school-age children in comparison with a placebo.[57]

Ipratroprium bromide (Atrovent [Boehringer Ingelheim Ltd., Ridgefield, CT]) is a new anticholinergic agent that is not yet released in the United States. Aerosolized ipratropium bromide was shown to produce bronchodilatation in 40% of infants under 18 months,[57a] the age group which beta agonists are relatively less effective. Nebulized ipratroprium bromie (250 μg) produced the same amount of bronchdilatation as 5 mg of nebulized albuterol in a group of pre-school-age asthmatics.[58]

Further studies are needed to establish the place of anticholinergics in the treatment of childhood asthma.

### Corticosteroids (Table 22-7)

In children, as in adults, corticosteroids are uniquely able to reverse the bronchodilator unresponsive component of airways obstruction by mechanisms that are not clearly understood. Corticosteroids have been shown to restore beta-adrenergic responsiveness within an hour after an IV dose[59] and to increase the $PaO_2$ in hypoxic children within 3 hours of administration.[60] Tenacious sputum attenuates, and mucosal edema is reduced. Therefore, corticosteroids are essential for treatment of the unresponsive airway obstruction characteristically seen in status asthmaticus and in patients ill enough to need hospitalization. No childhood asthmatic in status asthmaticus should be denied treatment with appropriate doses of corticosteroids because of a fear of inducing adrenal suppression or growth retardation. Short-term (less than 2 weeks) use of parenteral or oral corticosteroids rarely causes serious toxicity, although hypokalemia, mood alterations, weight gain, and GI discomfort can occur. Endogenous adrenal function will be suppressed by long-term daily administration of even low doses of corticosteroids (prednisone $<5$ mg/m$^2$ daily) in children,[61] and frequently there are serious adverse effects such as growth suppression, osteoporosis, cushingoid appearance, and subcapsular cataracts. Daily administration of corticosteroids in children thus must be employed for the shortest possible time to minimize these complications.

Chronic airway obstruction unresponsive to bronchodilators (theophylline and beta-adrenergic agents) in children as in adults must be treated with corticosteroids to restore beta-receptor "permissiveness." Short-acting prednisone is the preferred oral corticosteroid, although prednisolone and methylprednisolone (which are more expensive) are acceptable alternatives. Prednisone is now also available as a syrup (Liquid Pred [Muro Pharmaceutical, Inc. Tewksbury, MA] 5 mg per 5 ml) which possesses comparable bioavailability and earlier peak and higher first hour plasma prednisolone concentrations than the tablet.[61a] Dexamethasone suspension, although available, should be avoided because of its longer half-life and the unpredictable dose in a teaspoon of suspension. Enough prednisone should be given to induce a maximal therapeutic response as quickly as possible. Oral prednisone 1 to 2 mg/kg daily in two doses is usually sufficient to reverse the acute symptoms within 24–72 hours in outpatients, but larger doses or parenteral methylprednisolone (Solumedrol) given more frequently (Table 22-7) are generally necessary during status asthmaticus in hospitalized children. Corticosteroids should not be discontinued until the child becomes asymptomatic, and preferably not until spirometry returns to normal. Tapering of the dose to prevent adrenal insufficiency is not necessary if a corticosteroid has been given for only 4–5 days, but tapering may be essential in many patients to prevent recurrence of asthma symptoms. Prednisone should be given once daily before 8 A.M. during this tapering phase, which may last 7–10 days. If longer periods of daily prednisone are needed to prevent relapse, other regimens, including alternate-morning predisone, aerosol corticosteroids, or cromolyn, should be utilized.

Alternate-day steroid therapy refers to the administration of a single dose of a short-acting corticosteroid (prednisone, prednisolone, or methylprednisolone) every 48 hours, preferably before 8 A.M. This dosage schedule has been shown to cause minimal adrenal suppression and to reduce adverse steroid effects while maintaining good control of the bronchospasm.[62] A recent report suggests that there is no steroid-induced growth suppression in most childhood asthmatics who require and optimally use alternate-day corticosteroids for prolonged periods.[63] The average suppression of growth in children who received alternate-day or intermittent steroid treatment did not differ from that of asthmatics of comparable severity who did not receive steroids. However, children receiving low doses of alternate-day prednisone (mean dose 9.0 mg every other day) demonstrated more rapid growth than did those children receiving higher alternate-day dosage (mean dose of 30 mg).[64] These data may need to be reinterpreted in light of the documented delayed maturation of severe non-steroid-dependent asthmatics[38] since the group with the higher alternate-day steroid dose was 2 years older, approaching adolescence. If the adolescent growth spurt were delayed, there might be an apparent suppression of growth in early adolescence unrelated to corticosteroid dosage. Substitution of an alternate-day for a daily steroid regimen (mean dose 17 mg qod) did not induce a growth spurt even after 2 years of treatment, and children whose therapy was changed from a daily to an alternate-day prednisone regimen sometimes exhibited prolonged suppression (more than 4–6 months) of adrenal cortical function.[65] However, resting plasma cortisol levels became indistinguishable from those of a non-steroid-treated group between 1 and 2 months after alternate-day treatment was finally discontinued. Alternate-day prednisone treatment with doses of 20 mg or below does not appear to increase the risk of posterior-subcapsular cataracts,[66] but daily doses of 10 mg or more for longer than 1 year markedly increases the risk (7 of 17 patients).[67] Early cataracts have been shown to regress after patients were switched to aerosol steroids or after reduction of the daily dose of prednisone to below 10 mg.[67]

During treatment with inhaled corticosteroids such as beclomethasone dipropionate and flunisolide, oral steroid dependence can decrease, and suppressed adrenal-pituitary function can be restored in asthmatic adults. Beclomethasone 400 μg/day (about 10 puffs) is also effective in children above 6 years of age with steroid-dependent or severe non-steroid-dependent asthma. Its value in maintenance treatment has been demonstrated by improved spirometry, reduced frequency of asthma attacks, and decreased hospitalization during treatment periods in excess of 5 years.[68] Several studies have reported that adrenal function is normal with these doses of beclomethasone in children.[69,70] More recently Wyatt et al.[71] noted that inhaled beclomethasone at slightly higher doses (mean dose 550 μg/day or about 14 puffs) suppressed hypothalmic-pituitary-adrenal function to about the same degree as did alternate-day prednisone (mean dose 33 mg qod). The combination of beclomethasone and alternate-day prednisone was additive in suppression of adrenal function.[71] A recent study noted a dose of beclomethasone dipropionate of ≤13 μg/kg daily in childhood will not affect adrenal function.[71a] As with alternate-day prednisone, inhaled beclomethasone should be tapered to the lowest effective dose. Many childhood asthmatics are able to reduce total daily dosage below 200 μg (5 puffs) per day after the illness has been controlled. If an inhaled bronchodilator is given 5 minutes before the administration of beclomethasone, there is probably better delivery of the inhaled steroid to the peripheral airways, which may increase its effectiveness. Inhaled corticosteroids have the same drawbacks in childhood as in adults. With proper technique of administration, however, inhaled beclomethasone dipropionate, like alternate-day prednisone, is an effective form of treatment for children whose asthma is incompletely controlled with cromolyn and bronchodilators. Theophylline should not be discontinued when asthma symptoms are controlled on either of these prophylactic steroid regimens, since theophylline has been shown to reduce the requirement for corticosteroids and inhaled beta-adrenergic agents, and to improve spirometry in asthmatic children receiving maintenance steroid therapy.[72] Neither alternate-day prednisone nor inhaled corticosteroids should be used during exacerbations of asthma. Daily prednisone or its equivalent must be employed, and inhaled beclomethasone and cromolyn by spinhaler may need to be discontinued if they irritate the tracheobronchial tree and lead to increased asthma symptoms.

The decision to use alternate-day prednisone or inhaled beclomethasone during childhood must be based on individual considerations. Those children with obesity, diabetes, and immunologic disorders, or those with cushingism and other side effects might be excellent candidates for inhaled beclomethasone dipropionate. Children who are unable to inhale medication properly, are from impoverished families, or respond poorly to inhaled corticosteroids will probably do better on alternate-day prednisone.

Other methods have been explored to deliver topical corticosteroids to children below 5 years of age, who are usually unable to use a metered-dose inhaler. Freigang[73] reported the successful treatment of 67 severe asthmatic children between 1 and 5 years of age for at least 1 year with beclomethasone (maintenance dosage 200–300 μg/day) delivered by a special inhalational device consisting of a 1-liter plastic aerosol reservoir attached at one end to a face mask and at the other to the beclomethasone aerosol canister. After 2 puffs are delivered, the metered canister is replaced with a one-way valve, and the child inhales the medication as an aerosol through the face mask.[73] The recent development of other extension devices (ie: Aerochamber [Trudell Medical, Canada]) may be helpful in this age group[73a]

Flunisolide, a synthetic corticosteroid with potent topical anti-inflammatory activity, has been shown to be an effective treatment for asthma in adults and children. Asthmatic children who were not receiving steroids improved during an 8-week period when they were given flunisolide 1 mg/day by a metered-dose inhaler, and there was no evidence of adrenal suppression.[74] In steroid-dependent asthmatic children, 1 mg daily of inhaled flunisolide for 14 weeks reduced the requirement for oral steroids without suppressing adrenal function.[75] Any absorbed flunisolide is rapidly metabolized; thus there is little systemic exposure to the drug.[76] Flunisolide is now available as a solution for intranasal administration (250 $\mu$g/ml). Although not approved for nebulized use, flunisolide may be valuable for the treatment of early childhood asthma when given in aerosol form by a compressor-driven device. We have been encouraged by our results using 50–150 $\mu$g of nebulized flunisolide three times daily in asthmatics below 5 years of age, but long-term follow-up will be needed before precise recommendations can be given. Parenthetically, adult steroid-dependent asthmatics unable to inhale beclomethasone correctly or in whom the drug has led to incessant cough may improve with nebulized flunisolide 250 $\mu$g three or four times daily.

### Miscellaneous Agents

Oxygen is all too often omitted in the treatment of children with acute asthma, although hypoxemia always occurs during these episodes. Administration of oxygen at 3–4 liters/min by a face mask or nasal cannula is generally adequate for the typical asthmatic attack. Higher concentrations of oxygen may be delivered by venturi masks or croup tents if necessary.

Antihistamines such as hydroxyzine and chlorpheniramine that can block histamine-induced bronchospasm and the immediate bronchospastic response to antigen may deserve a trial, particularly in the patient rendered irritable by the usual theophylline and beta-adrenergic preparations. Antihistamines need not be avoided for fear of "drying out" the tracheobronchial tree, however. Recently a broad spectrum of antihistamines adversely affected spirometry in 10 selected asthmatic children.[76a] The great value of controlling upper respiratory complaints in the asthmatic is discussed in Chapter 21.

Expectorants have no place in the treatment of childhood asthma. Iodides can cause goiter and hypothyroidism, and acetylcysteine may induce bronchospasm. Antimicrobial agents are ineffective in most episodes of acute asthma unless there is clinical evidence of bacterial disease. Sedatives should be avoided during acute asthma in childhood as irritability may be a symptom of impending respiratory failure rather than emotional lability.

*Immunotherapy.* There have been only four placebo-controlled studies demonstrating that allergen immunotherapy can reduce symptoms or the response to bronchial provocation in childhood asthma. When the results of these studies were pooled, 122 of 162 or 75% of the allergen-treated group and 37 of 129 or 29% of the placebo group improved.[77] Despite the small number of subjects studied and the potential risk of major adverse reactions, immunotherapy has been rather indiscriminately recommended for asthmatic children, often before environmental control measures and appropriate medications have been instituted. The indications, risks, and relative benefits of immunotherapy of IgE-mediated asthma are discussed in Chapter 15. A paradox inherent in immunotherapy that becomes apparent to any critical allergist is that the severe asthmatic benefits least whereas those with milder asthma do not need it because they respond to environmental and pharmacologic measures.

## Complications in Childhood Asthma

The right middle-lobe syndrome, characterized by recurrent or persistent atelectasis of the right middle lobe, is common in childhood asthmatics. The condition develops by 1–2 years of age, but the diagnosis is usually delayed for several years. It is twice as common in girls as in boys, and 70% of the cases are atopic. Cough and wheeze are invariable symptoms. Seventy percent of patients show inspiratory rales, and 50% have recurrent pneumonias. Plain chest x-rays are invariably abnormal during acute exacerbations. Eighty percent of patients have abnormal sinus x-rays, bronchography, if performed, is abnormal in 90%. Medical treatment must be aggressive and should include bronchodilators, postural drainage with physical therapy, appropriate antibiotics (after culture and gram stain of sputum), and often corticosteroids. Radiologic improvement is usually seen within 4–6 weeks, but total resolution may take several months. Bronchoscopy and bronchography are reserved for the child who has not responded to medical treatment or when surgical intervention is considered. The typical findings are compressing lymph nodes, an abnormally small right middle-lobe bronchus, purulent secretions, and bronchiectasis.[78]

Atelectasis of lung areas other than the right middle lobe is not infrequent. Up to 20% of hospitalized asthmatic children demonstrate atelectasis radiographically. Persistent atelectasis may result from foreign bodies, anatomic defects, mucus plugging, or enlarged bronchial lymph nodes. Bronchoscopy is rarely necessary since in 95% of the cases aggressive treatment of the underlying asthma will eliminate mucus plugging and the atelectatic regions will reexpand.

Allergic bronchopulmonary aspergillosis (ABPA) is an infrequent complication of childhood asthma. However, up to 11% of children with cystic fibrosis, usually those with severe disease, may fulfill the diagnostic criteria for ABPA.[79]

Growth retardation is characteristic of severe childhood asthma. Frequently there are thoracic deformities, including barrel chest, pigeon breast, and Harrison's groove. Successful treatment may reverse these abnormalities within a year or two. The severely asthmatic child usually has a very delayed growth spurt at 18 or 19 years of age.

Many children with acute asthma vomit incessantly because of coughing and excessive mucus secretion. Such vomiting makes it difficult to give oral medications and may lead to dehydration, thus worsening the asthma. Nebulized beta-adrenergic agents may provide adequate bronchodilation at these times. Antiemetic suppositories may reduce vomiting, but they must be used cautiously to avoid excessive sedation. Aggressive treatment during the prodome before the asthma becomes severe generally will prevent the vomiting episodes. Occasionally a few hours of IV hydration will reverse the vomiting-dehydration cycle and avoid the need for hospitalization.

Children with severe asthma lost 2½ times as much time from school as their healthy contemporaries; thus one of the potential complications of the disease is poor school performance. These problems can be mitigated with appropriate tutoring and special physical education.

Respiratory failure[80,81] occurs in about 1% (13 of 1255) of all children admitted to the hospital with acute asthma (mean age 4 years). Viral infection was suspected or proved in 10 of the 13 episodes. Previous hospitalizations were frequent among these patients, averaging five per patient. Respiratory failure develops rapidly in childhood; in 11 of 12 of these children, wheezing had appeared only 2–18 hours before admission.[17] Adolescent asthmatics are also vulnerable to respiratory failure because of their denial of symptoms, abuse of inhaled bronchodilators, and delay in seeking medical assistance.

## PERSPECTIVES ON FUTURE DEVELOPMENTS
## IN CHILDHOOD ALLERGIC DISEASE

Several studies have suggested, although non-conclusively, that environmental engineering that minimizes allergen exposure at critical times during infancy will prevent, delay the onset, or reduce the severity of allergic disorders in childhood. There are several theoretical reasons for IgE mediated disorders being amenable to prevention efforts:

1.  Allergic disorders are common and inheritable and occur mainly in identifiable populations.
2.  Individuals likely to have allergic offspring can be identified by simple and inexpensive assays. Specific IgE reactivity can be rapidly determined in men and nonpregnant women by allergy skin tests. In pregnant women, elevated serum IgE (50 U/ml) alone or low IgE with one positive radioallergosorbent (RAST) would strongly suggest atopy.
3.  At-risk infants can be identified at birth. Elevated IgE levels in the umbilical cord blood have been associated with subsequent development of atopic illnesses, and the serum IgE can be periodically measured during infancy.

A practical approach to prevention that is now undergoing investigation includes the following measures. The mother avoids milk products and eggs during her last trimester and lactation and breast-feeds the infant for 4–6 months. Highly allergenic foods are avoided during infancy, and inhaled allergens avoided as completely as possible throughout life. We are now conducting a prospective study of these measures, comparing the treated group with a control group of at-risk infants receiving a commercial milk formula without any special dietary restrictions on their mothers. Confirmation of the results of a previous open trial may have major impact on the entire approach to the at-risk atopic newborn.[82]

## REFERENCES

1.  Weiss ST, Tager IB, Speizer FE, et al: Persistent wheeze: Its relationship to respiratory illness, cigarette smoking, and level of pulmonary function in a population sample of children. Am Rev Respir Dis 122:697–707, 1980
2.  Blair H: Natural history of childhood asthma. Arch Dis Childh 52:613–619, 1977
3.  Martin AJ, McLennan LA, Landau LI, et al: Natural history of childhood asthma to adult life. Br Med J 1:1397–1400, 1980
4.  Kuzemko JA: Natural history of childhood asthma. J Pediatr 97:886–892, 1980
5.  Broder I, Higgins MW, Matthews KP, et al: Epidemiology of asthma and allergic rhinitis in a total community, Tecumseh, Michigan. J Allergy Clin Immunol 54:100–110, 1974
6.  Hogg JC, Williams J, Richardson JB, et al: Age as a factor in the distribution of lower airway conductance and in the pathologic anatomy of obstructive lung disease. New Engl J Med 282:1283–1287, 1970
7.  Reid L: Pathological changes in asthma, in Clark TJH, Godfrey S (Eds): Asthma. Philadelphia, Saunders, 1977, pp 79–95.
8.  Shannon DC: Asthma in children. Clin Notes Respir Dis 15:3–9, 1976
9.  Lenney W, Milner AD: At what age do bronchodilator drugs work? Arch Dis Childh 53:532–535, 1978
10.  Tal A, Bavilski C, Yohai D, et al: Dexamethasone and salbutamol in the treatment of acute wheezing in infants. Pediatrics 71:13–18, 1983

11. Bryan AC, Mansell AL, Levison H: Development of the mechanical properties of the respiratory system, in Hodson WA (Ed): Development of the Lung, vol 6. New York, Marcel Dekker, 1977, p 445

12. Macklin CC: Alveolar pores and their significance in the human lung. Arch Pathol 21:202–216, 1936

13. Muller NL, Bryan AC: Chest wall mechanics and respiratory muscles in infants. Pediatr Clin N Am 26:503–516, 1979

14. Keens IG, Bryan AC, Levison H, et al: Developmental pattern of muscle fibre types in human ventilatory muscles. J Appl Physiol 44:909–913, 1978

15. Tabachnik E, Levison H: Infantile bronchial asthma. J Allergy Clin Immunol 67:339–347, 1981

16. Minor TE, Baker JW, Dick EC, et al: Greater frequency of viral respiratory infections in asthmatic children as compared with their nonasthmatic siblings. J Pediatr 85:472–477, 1974

17. Simpson H, Mitchell I, Inglis JM, et al: Severe ventilatory failure in asthma in children. Arch Dis Childh 53:714–721, 1978

18. Horn MEC, Reed SE, Taylor P: Role of viruses and bacteria in acute wheezy bronchitis in childhood: A study of sputum. Arch Dis Childh 54:587–592, 1979

19. Empey DW, Laitinen LA, Jacobs L, et al: Mechanisms of bronchial hyperactivity in normal subjects after upper respiratory tract infection. Am Rev Respir Dis 113:131–139, 1976

20. Aquilina AT, Hall WJ, Douglas GR, et al: Airway reactivity in subjects with viral upper respiratory tract infections: The effects of exercise and cold air. Am Rev Respir Dis 122:3–9, 1980

21. Welliver RC, Wong DT, Sun M, et al: The development of respiratory synctial virus-specific IgE and the release of histamine in nasopharyngeal secretions after infection. N Engl J Med 305:841–846, 1981

22. Gurwitz D, Mindorff C, Levison H: Increased incidence of bronchial reactivity in children with a history of bronchiolitis. J Pediatr 98:551–558, 1981

23. Sims DG, Gardner PS, Weightman D, et al: Atopy does not predispose to RSV bronchiolitis or postbronchiolitic wheezing. Br Med J 282:2086–2088, 1981

24. Henderson FW, Collier AM, Clyde WA, et al: Respiratory-synctial-virus infections, reinfections and immunity. New Engl J Med 300:530–534, 1979

25. Kattan M, Keens TG, Lapierre JG, et al: Pulmonary function abnormalities in symptom-free children after bronchiolitis. Pediatrics 59:683–688, 1977

26. Gurwitz D, Corey M, Levison H: Pulmonary function and bronchial reactivity in children after croup. Am Rev Respir Dis 122:95–99, 1980

27. Zach M, Erben A, Olinsky A: Croup, recurrent croup, allergy and airways hyperreactivity. Arch Dis Childh 56:336–341, 1981

28. Zach MS, Schnall RP, Landau LI: Upper and lower airway hyperactivity in recurrent croup. Am Rev Respir Dis 121:979–983, 1980

29. Kawabori I, Pierson WR, Conquest LL, et al: Incidence of exercise-induced asthma in children. J Allergy Clin Immunol 58:447–455, 1976

30. Fitch KD, Morton AR, Blanksby BA: Effects of swimming training on children with asthma. Arch Dis Childh 51:190–194, 1976

31. Rachelefsky GS, Coulson A, Siegel SC, et al: Aspirin intolerance in chronic childhood asthma detected by oral challenge. Pediatrics 56:443–448, 1975

32. Herst JJ: Gastroesophageal reflux. J Pediatr 98:859–870, 1981

33. Berquist WE, Rachelefsky GS, Kadden M, et al: Gastroesophageal reflux associated recurrent pneumonia and chronic asthma in children. Pediatrics 68:29–35, 1981

34. Cloutier MM, Loughlin GM: Chronic cough in children: A manifestation of airway hyperactivity. Pediatrics 67:6–12, 1981

35. Hannaway PS, Hopper DK: Cough variant asthma in children. JAMA 247:206–208, 1982

36. Shapiro GG, Furukawa CT, Pierson WE, et al: Methacholine bronchial challenge in children. J Allergy Clin Immunol 69:365–369, 1982

37. McNicol KN, Williams HB: Spectrum of asthma in children. I. Clinical and physiological components. Br Med J 4:7–11, 1973

38. Hauspie R, Susanne C, Alexander F: Maturational delay and temporal growth retardation in asthmatic boys. J Allergy Clin Immunol 59:200–206, 1977

39. Loren ML, Leung PK, Cooley RL, et al: Irreversibility of obstructive changes in severe asthma in childhood. Chest 74:126–129, 1978

40. Commey JOO, Levison H: Physical signs in childhood asthma. Pediatrics 58:537–541, 1976

41. Eggleston PA, Ward BH, Pierson WE, Bierman CW: Radiographic abnormalities in acute asthma in children. Pediatrics 54:442–449, 1974

42. Frommell GT, Rothenberg R, Wang S, et al: Chlamydial infection of mothers and their infants. J Pediatr 95:28–32, 1979

43. May CD, Bock SA: Adverse reactions to food due to hypersensitivity, in Middleton E Jr, Reed CE, Ellis E (Eds): Allergy: Principles and Practice. St. Louis, Mosby, 1978, pp 1159–1171

43a. Zeiger RS, Jalowayski A, Schatz M: Chronic rhinitis: only half a diagnosis. Diagnosis 5:1–7, 1983

44. Brooks LJ, Cropp JA: Theophylline therapy in bronchiolitis. Am J Dis Childh 135:934–936, 1981

45. Weinberger M, Hendeles L, Ahrens R: Pharmacologic management of reversible obstructive airways disease. Med Clin N Am 65:579–613, 1980

46. Ellis EF: Theophylline and derivatives, in Middleton E Jr, Reed CE, Ellis E (Eds): Allergy: Principles and Practice. St. Louis, Mosby, 1978, pp 434–453

47. Arwood LL, Dasta JF, Friedman C: Placental transfer of theophylline: Two case reports. Pediatrics 63:844–846, 1979

48. Rachelefsky GS, Katz RM, Siegel SC: Albuterol syrup in the treatment of the young asthmatic child. Ann Allergy 57:143–146, 1981

49. Michaelson ED, Silva GT, Forrest TR, et al: Effects of oral terbutaline in children with bronchial asthma. J Allergy Clin Immunol 51:365–369, 1978

50. Sackner MA, Silva G, Zucker C, et al: Long-term effects of metaproterenol in asthmatic children. Am Rev Respir Dis 115:945–953, 1977

51. Galant SP, Groncy CE, Duriseti S, et al: The effect of metaproterenal in chronic asthmatic children receiving therapeutic doses of theophylline. J Allergy Clin Immunol 61:73–78, 1978

52. Garra B, Shapiro GG, Dorsett C, et al: A double-blind evaluation of the use of nebulized metaproterenol and isoproterenol in hospitalized asthmatic children and adolescents. J Allergy Clin Immunol 60:63–68, 1977

53. Schwartz AL, Lipton JM, Warburton D, et al: Management of acute asthma in childhood. Am J Dis Childh 134:474–476, 1980

54. Konig P: Conflicting viewpoints about treatment of asthma with cromolyn: A review of the literature. Ann Allergy 43:293–296, 1979

55. Lenney W, Milner AD: Nebulized sodium cromoglycate in the preschool wheezy child. Arch Dis Child 53:474–476, 1978

55a. Hiller EJ, Milner AD, Lenney W: Nebulized sodium cromoglycate in young asthmatic children. Arch Dis Child 52:875–876, 1977

55b. Glass J, Archer LNJ, Adams W, Simpson H: Nebulized cromoglycate theophylline and placebo in preschool asthmatic children. Arch Dis Child 56:648–651, 1981

55c. Newth CJL, Newth CV, Turner JAP: Comparison of nebulized sodium cromoglycate and oral theophylline in controlling symptoms of chronic asthma in pre-school children: A double blind study. Aust N Z J Med 12:232–238, 1982

55d. Mellon MH, Harden K, Zeiger RS: The effectiveness and safety of nebulizer cromolyn solution in the young childhood asthmatic. Immunol Allergy Practice 4:168–172, 1982

56. Hemstreet MP: Atropine nebulization—simple and safe. Ann Allergy 44:138–139, 1980

57. Hutchison A, Olinsky A, Landau L: Long term atropine in chronic severe childhood asthma. J Aust Paediatr 16:267–269, 1980

57a. Hodges IGC, Groggins RC, Milner AD, Stokes GM: Bronchodilator effect of inhaled ipratropium bromide in wheezy toddlers. Arch Dis Child 56:729–731 1981

58. Groggins RC, Milner AD, Stokes GM: Bronchodilator effects of clemastine, ipratropium bromide, and salbutamol in preschool children with asthma. Arch Dis Childh 56:342–344, 1981

59. Ellul-Micallef R, Fenech FF: Effect of intravenous prednisolone in asthmatics with diminished adrenergic responsiveness. Lancet 2:1269–1270, 1975

60. Pierson WE, Bierman CW, Kelley VC: A double blind trial of corticosteroid therapy in status asthmaticus. Pediatrics 54:282–288, 1974

61. Van Metre TE Jr, Pinkerton HL Jr: Growth suppression in asthmatic children receiving prolonged therapy with prednisone and methyl prednisolone. J Allergy 30:103–113, 1959

61a. Georgitis JW, Flesher KA & Szefler SJ: Bioavailability assessment of a liquid prednisone preparation. J All Clin Immun 70:243–247, 1982

62. Falliers CJ, Chai H, Molk L, et al: Pulmonary and adrenal effects of alternate-day corticosteroid therapy. J Allergy Clin Immunol 49:156–166, 1972

63. Siegel SC, Goldberg M, Richards W, et al: Effects of alternate-day corticosteroid therapy on linear growth in children with intractable asthma. Israel J Med Sci 6:743, 1970 (abstr)

64. Reimer LG, Morris HG, Ellis EF: Growth of asthmatic children during treatment with alternate-day steroids. J Allergy Clin Immunol 55:224–231, 1975

65. Morris HG, Neuman I, Ellis EF: Plasma steroid concentrations during alternate-day treatment with prednisone. J Allergy Clin Immunol 54:350–358, 1974

66. Sevel D, Weinberg MB, Van Niekerk CH: Lenticular complications of long-term steroid therapy in children with asthma and eczema. J Allergy Clin Immunol 60:215–217, 1977

67. Rooklin AR, Lampert SI, Jaeger EA, et al: Posterior subcapsular cataracts in steroid-requiring asthmatic children. J Allergy Clin Immunol 63:383–386, 1979

68. Godfrey S, Balfour-Lynn L, Tooley M: A three to five year follow-up of the use of the aerosol steroid, beclomethasone dipropionate, in childhood asthma. J Allergy Clin Immunol 62:335–339, 1978

69. Klein R, Waldman D, Kershnar H, et al: Treatment of chronic asthma with beclomethasone dipropionate aerosol: I. A double-blind cross-over trial in nonsteroid-dependent patients, Pediatrics 60:7–13, 1977

70. Kershnar H, Klein R, Waldman D, et al: Treatment of chronic childhood asthma with beclomethasone dipropionate aerosols: II. Effect on pituitary-adrenal function after substitution for oral corticosterods. Pediatrics 62:189–197, 1978

71. Wyatt R, Wascheck J, Weinberger M, et al: Effects of inhaled beclomethasone dipropionate and alternate-day prednisone on pituitary-adrenal function in children with chronic asthma. New Engl J Med 299:1387–1392, 1978

71a. Sherman B, Weinberger M, Chen-Walden H, Wendt H: Further studies of the effects of inhaled glucocorticoids on pituitary-adrenal function in healthy adults. J Allergy Clin Immunol 69:208–212, 1982

72. Nassif EG, Weinberger M, Thompson R, et al: The value of maintenance theophylline in steroid-dependent asthma. New Engl J Med 304:71–75, 1981

73. Freigang B: Long term follow-up of infants and children treated with beclomethasone aerosol by a special inhalation device. Ann Allergy 45:13–17, 1980

73a. Hodges IGC, Milner AD, Stokes GM: Assessment of a new device for delivering aerosol drugs to asthmatic children. Arch Dis Child 56:787–800, 1981

74. Meltzer EO, Kemp JP, Orgel HA, Izu, AE: Flunisolide aerosol for treatment of severe, chronic asthma in steroid-independent children. Pediatrics 69:340–345, 1982

75. Shapiro GG, Izu AE, Furukawa CT, Pierson WE, Bierman CW: Short-term double-blind evaluation of flunisolide aerosol for steroid-dependent asthmatic children and adolescents. Chest 80:671–675, 1981

76. Chaplin MD, Rooks W, Swenson EW, et al: Flunisolide metabolism and dynamics of a metabolite. Clin Pharmacol Ther 27:402–413, 1980

76a. Schuller DE: The spectrum of antihistamines adversely affecting pulmonary function in asthmatic children. Abstracted, J Allergy Clin Immunol 71:Part 2 147, 1983

77. Zeiger RS, Schatz M: Immunotherapy of atopic disorders: Present state of the art and future perspectives. Med Clin N Am 65:987–1012, 1981

78. Dees SC, Spock A: Right middle lobe syndrome in children. JAMA 197:8–14, 1966

79. Nelson LA, Callerame ML, Schwartz RH: Aspergillosis and atopy in cystic fibrosis. Am Rev Respir Dis 120:863–873, 1979

80. Pearlman DS, Bierman CW: Asthma (bronchial asthma, reactive airways disorder), in Bierman CW, Pearlman DS (Eds): Allergic Diseases of Infancy, Childhood, and Adolescence. Philadelphia, Saunders, 1980, pp 581–604

81. Simons FER: Asthma in children. Semin Respir Med 1:147–166, 1979

82. Schatz M, Zeiger RS, Mellon M, et al: The course and management of asthma and allergic disease during pregnancy, in Middleton E, Ellis G, Reed CE (ed): *Allergy: Principles and Practice*, St. Louis, Mosby, 1983, pp 935–986

## 23

MICHAEL SCHATZ

# Asthma and Pregnancy

Asthma complicates at least 1% of pregnancies[1] and is probably the most common single medical condition that occurs during pregnancy. When asthma and pregnancy coexist, several important questions emerge. What effect does asthma have on the course and outcome of pregnancy? What effect does pregnancy have on the course of asthma? What is the optimal way to manage asthma during pregnancy and lactation, considering the welfare of both the mother and the baby? This chapter attempts to provide practical answers to these questions, based on information currently available. The reader is also referred to several other recent reviews of this subject.[2-4]

## PHYSIOLOGY AND IMMUNOLOGY OF NORMAL PREGNANCY

When considering any medical condition during pregnancy, one must recognize the normal physiologic changes that occur during pregnancy and the possible effects of these changes on the illness. There are a number of hormonal and other biochemical changes that occur during pregnancy associated with physiologic and immunologic changes that could influence the course of gestational asthma.

The hormonal changes associated with normal pregnancy are summarized in Tables 23-1 and 23-2 and are reviewed elsewhere.[5] The potential immunosuppressive effects of human chorionic gonadotropin and possibly progesterone may be relevant to intrapartum immunologic disease. Progesterone also appears to be responsible for the increased ventilation and decreased airways resistance that occur during pregnancy. The increased free cortisol during pregnancy might be beneficial in patients with asthma. However, little is known about the actual impact of these changes on gestational asthma.

The pulmonary physiologic changes during pregnancy have been reviewed recently[6] (see also Table 23-3). Ventilation increases out of proportion to the increased oxygen consumption and metabolic needs of pregnancy, so that blood gases during normal pregnancy show a partially compensated respiratory alkolosis (Table 23-4). These normal gestational blood gases have two main implications relevant to acute gestational asthma.

The Kaiser-Permanente prospective study of asthma during pregnancy has been supported in part by a grant from the William H. Rorer-Dooner Laboratories. I would also like to thank Susette Caggiano for her excellent secretarial assistance.

**Table 23-1**
**Placental Hormone Changes During Pregnancy**

| Hormone | Time Course | Functions |
|---|---|---|
| Human chorionic gonadotrapin | Detectable: 1 day postimplantation | Luteotrophic: early pregnancy |
| | Peak: 60–90 days, plateau thereafter | Regulates fetal steroid production |
| | | Thyroid-stimulating activity |
| | | Immunosuppressive effects |
| Human chorionic somatomammotropin | Detectable: early first TM* | Metabolic effects Growth-hormone-like contrainsulin effects |
| | Rises: 20–36 weeks, plateau thereafter | |

*trimester.

**Table 23-2**
**Steroid Hormone Changes During Pregnancy**

| Hormone | Time Course | Functions |
|---|---|---|
| Progesterone | Rises steadily from early gestation to term | Relaxation of smooth muscle |
| | | Increased ventilatory response |
| | | Immunosuppressive effects (?) |
| Estrogen | Rises steadily from early gestation to term | Increased uteroplacental blood flow |
| | | Softening of cervical connective tissue |
| Cortisol | | |
| CBG* | Increases with increasing gestation | |
| Total | Increases with increasing gestation | |
| Free | Small increase with increasing gestation | |

*cortisol binding globulin.

**Table 23-3**
**Established Pulmonary Physiologic Changes During Pregnancy**

Ventilation
    Increased minute ventilation
    Increased alveolar ventilation
    Increased oxygen consumption

Lung Volumes
    Increased tidal volume
    Decreased functional residual capacity (FRC)
        Decreased expiratory reserve volume
        Decreased residual volume
    Closing volume nearer to FRC
    Normal vital capacity, total lung capacity

Airway mechanics
    Decreased total pulmonary and airway resistance
    Normal forced expiratory volume in 1 second ($FEV_1$)
    Normal dynamic compliance
    Normal maximal midexpiratory flow rate

First, the changes in blood gases due to acute asthma will be superimposed on the "normal" respiratory alkalosis of pregnancy. Thus a $PCO_2 > 35$ or a $PO_2$ of less than 70 mm Hg associated with asthma will represent more dire circumstances during pregnancy than will similar blood gases in the nongravid state. Second, maternal $PO_2$ and pH are major determinants of fetal oxygenation so that hypoxia, alkalosis, and especially the combination of the two can lead to impaired fetal oxygenation. Therefore, it is very important to adequately treat or, better still, to prevent severe asthma during pregnancy. In addition, oxygen therapy during acute gestational asthma must be sufficient to prevent fetal hypoxia.

The distribution of the static subdivisions of lung volume changes during pregnancy. The change of most relevance to asthma is the increased proximity of the closing volume to the functional residual capacity (FRC). If the small airways close at a lung volume near the FRC (i.e., during tidal breathing), there is decreased ventilation of the dependent regions of the lung and the alveolar–arterial $PO_2$ gradient will increase. This change during normal pregnancy may intensify the low ventilation–perfusion ratios and the

**Table 23-4**
**Blood Gases During Normal Pregnancy**

| Parameter | Change | Range |
|-----------|--------|-------|
| $PO_2$ | Increased | 106–108 mm Hg (1st trimester) |
| | | 101–104 mm Hg (3rd trimester) |
| $PCO_2$ | Decreased | 27–32 mm Hg |
| pH | Normal or slightly increased | 7.40–7.47 |
| Bicarbonate | Decreased | 18–21 meq/l |

**Table 23-5**
**Maternal Immunologic Changes During Pregnancy**

Hormonal
  Decreased IgG

  1.  Specific (viral)
        Total
            Dilutional
            Cord blood T-cell suppression

  IgE changes—variable

Cellular
  Lymphoid tissues—decreased size, cellularity, germinal centers

  Relative lymphopenia, absolute lymphocytosis

  Decreased in vitro responsiveness—phytohemagglutin, mixed lymphocyte culture, rubella

    Isolated lymphocytes
    Suppressive serum factors
      IgG antibody
      Immune complexes
      alpha-Fetoprotein
      Pregnancy hormones
    Cord blood lymphocyte suppression

resulting hypoxemia that occur as a result of bronchial obstruction when acute asthma complicates pregnancy.

During normal pregnancy the airways resistance falls, which implies a decrease in the bronchomotor tone in large central airways. This should be beneficial in patients with asthma, but since there are no concomitant changes in the resistance of the small peripheral airways, the alterations in large airway tone are probably insignificant clinically.

The immunologic changes associated with pregnancy are summarized in Table 23-5 and are reviewed in more detail elsewhere.[2,7] Most of these changes appear to be teliologically related to inhibiting maternal rejection of the histoincompatible fetus. One can only speculate on the possible relationships of these changes to gestational asthma. The decrease in humoral and cellular immune function could be important to asthma during pregnancy by causing increased susceptibility to respiratory infections that may trigger the asthma. Indeed, sinusitis has been reported to occur six times more commonly during

**Table 23-6**
**Increased Serum Mediators During Pregnancy**

Cyclic AMP
Cyclic GMP
Histamine
Histaminase
Prostaglandin F
Prostaglandin E (3rd trimester)

pregnancy than in the nongravid state.[8] Changes in total IgE during pregnancy may reflect changes in specific IgE antibody that could affect the course of allergic asthma during pregnancy. In a small study, those women with an increasing or unchanging IgE level tended to worsen during pregnancy, whereas those with a decreasing level during pregnancy (which was the pattern in normal controls) tended to improve or remain the same.[9] The increase during pregnancy of certain mediators in the serum (Table 23-6) also has a potential but as yet unidentified effect on the course of gestational allergies and asthma.

## EFFECT OF ASTHMA ON PREGNANCY

Asthma might have an unfavorable effect on pregnancy or on the fetus because of hypoxia, the medications required by the mother, or other associated factors. Two large retrospective studies suggest that asthma really does increase the risk of pregnancy (Table 23-7). Bahna and Bjerkedal[10] reported a statistically significant (1) increase in preterm births, (2) increase in low-birth-weight infants, (3) decrease in mean birth weight, (4) increase in neonatal mortality, and (5) increase in neonatal hypoxia in asthmatic pregnancies compared to pregnancies in women with no complicating medical illnesses. Gordon et al.[1] reported a statistically significant increase in perinatal mortality in infants of asthmatic mothers compared to the entire study population and found that women with severe asthma were particularly at risk of perinatal complications. The retrospective nature of these studies does not allow one to determine how well the asthma was controlled or how medications, genetic factors, or other relevant variables increased the risk of an adverse outcome in the asthmatic women in the two studies reported in Table 23-7.

Preliminary data from our Kaiser-Permanente Prospective Study of Asthma During

Table 23-7
Effect of Asthma on Pregnancy: Retrospective Studies

| Parameter | Bahna and Bjerkedal | | | Gordon et al. | | |
| --- | --- | --- | --- | --- | --- | --- |
| | Asthma | Control | Significance Value | Asthma | Control | Significance Value |
| Number of pregnancies | 381 | 112,530 | — | 277 | 30,861 | — |
| Preterm births | 7.4% | 5.0% | $p < .01$ | 14.4% | 18.0% | NS |
| Low-birth-weight infants | 7.1% | 3.7% | $p < .001$ | 15.2% | 11.4% | NS |
| Mean birth weight | 3,399.9 | 3,496.7 | $p < .001$ | | — | |
| Perinatal mortality | 2.6% | 1.5% | NS* | 5.9% | 3.2% | $p < .05$ |
| Neonatal low Apgar score or hypoxia | 1.6% | 0.7% | $p < .05$ | 5.0% | 3.9% | NS |
| Congenital malformations | 5.0% | 3.9% | NS | | — | |

*not significant.

Pregnancy have been analyzed in 120 prospectively managed asthmatic women who were compared with matched controls. Asthmatic patients in this study had no more perinatal complications than did control women. These preliminary data suggest that if asthmatic women are identified early in pregnancy and if they are appropriately managed, they have no increased risk of important perinatal complications, but many more women must be studied to confirm this hypothesis.

## EFFECT OF PREGNANCY ON ASTHMA

Data in the literature suggest that the overall effect of pregnancy on the course of asthma varies from individual to individual.[9] In the first 120 asthmatic women in our Kaiser-Permanente Prospective Study of Asthma During Pregnancy, 28% improved, 29% remained unchanged, and 33% worsened during pregnancy. In the remaining 10%, the change in the course of their asthma during pregnancy could have been explained by identifiable factors other than pregnancy. The variable effect of pregnancy on the course of asthma appears to be more than merely random fluctuation in the natural course of the disease, since the changes with pregnancy may be dramatic and may revert rapidly back to the non-pregnant state after delivery. It seems likely that there are multiple biochemical, immunologic, physiologic, and psychological factors that may ameliorate or exacerbate asthma during pregnancy and that the importance of these factors varies from one individual to another. Presumably the net effect of these factors in the individual patient determines what influence, if any, pregnancy will have on the course of the asthma.

There are two factors that may help to predict how pregnancy will affect a woman's asthma: (1) the course of asthma is often consistent in an individual woman with each pregnancy (e.g., in one study of asthmatic women, the course of the asthma was similarly affected with each pregnancy in 63%[11]); and (2) the course of the asthma during pregnancy shows a correlation with the severity of the preexisting disease. Those women with moderate or severe asthma prior to pregnancy are more likely to worsen and less likely to improve during pregnancy than are women with milder disease.[9,11] However, although this general relationship between increased non-pregnant disease severity and increased likelihood of exacerbation during pregnancy may be valid, the not uncommon exceptions dictate that all patients with asthma during pregnancy must be monitored closely for a change in their clinical status so that the therapeutic regimen can be adjusted accordingly.

Several other observations can be made about the course of asthma during pregnancy. The change in course of gestational asthma in an individual patient is frequently obvious during the first trimester, especially when the asthma improves. Upper respiratory infections are probably the most common precipitant of severe exacerbations of asthma during pregnancy, and the peak incidence of flares appears to be between the 24th and 36th weeks of gestation. In contrast, asthma frequently improves during the few weeks prior to delivery and is generally quiescent during labor and delivery itself. Of the first 120 asthmatic women who delivered in the Kaiser-Permanente Prospective Study of Asthma During Pregnancy, 90% had no asthma symptoms at all during labor and delivery. Of the 12 patients who did, 6 required no treatment, 5 responded to inhaled bronchodilators, and only 1 required intravenous (IV) aminophylline. The antepartum asthma treatment program was continued during labor in all these patients.

## MANAGEMENT OF ASTHMA DURING PREGNANCY AND LACTATION

An obvious goal of asthma therapy during pregnancy is to prevent asthma so severe as to potentially cause fetal hypoxia. In addition, one should attempt to provide an acceptable level of comfort for the pregnant woman so as to prevent symptoms that could interfere with the pregnancy through an effect on eating, sleeping, or emotional well-being. The patient should be questioned and examined, and spirometry should be done frequently by physicians skilled in managing asthma in order to carry the patient safely and successfully through her pregnancy.

### Psychologic Management

Pregnancy represents a time of psychological vulnerability for virtually all women. Change in body image, the physical symptoms accompanying normal pregnancy, and various natural fears regarding the pregnancy and the developing fetus are major sources of psychological stress.[12] In the pregnant woman with asthma, these stresses may be especially important. First, in women whose asthma tends to worsen with stress, the stress of normal pregnancy may cause an exacerbation of symptoms. Conversely, the discomfort associated with asthma, especially if the symptoms interfere with sleep, may add substantially to the stress of normal pregnancy.

Asthma management during pregnancy must thus include certain psychological techniques in order to minimize psychological morbidity.[12] The patient must be allowed ample opportunity to express her fears and concerns, which should be therapeutic in itself. The patient should also be educated regarding asthma in general and the interrelationships of asthma and pregnancy. Such knowledge provides a sense of mastery over the frightening unknown and should reduce anxiety. Moreover, the medical physician should be an important source of support for the patient so that she will not feel that she must handle her illness alone. Regular visits and easy accessibility for unexpected problems should allow the medical physician to provide this support. Finally, the reassurance provided by all of these sources and measures will be helpful in reducing anxiety during pregnancy. In addition, the patient should be specifically reassured that the medical physician, the obstetrician, and the patient will work as a team to maximize the health of the mother and the baby.

### Immunologic Management

The first principle of immunologic therapy is avoidance, and this is particularly important during pregnancy, since avoidance procedures increase the likelihood of physical well-being without pharmacologic intervention. Full information on antigen and irritant avoidance should be given to the patient (see Chapter 19). The patient should be convinced that it is extremely unwise to experience symptoms (which may require medication) due to avoidable exposure during pregnancy when not only she, but also the baby stands to suffer.

Abortions associated with systemic reactions following antigen immunotherapy have been reported.[13] Aside from systemic reactions, allergen immunotherapy appears safe during pregnancy. A recent study of 121 pregnancies in 90 women receiving immunotherapy reported no increased incidence of abortions, fetal deaths, neonatal deaths, prematuri-ty, toxemia, or congenital malformations in the treated patients in comparison with the general population.[14] In addition, six women experienced systemic reactions in this series without abortions or infant abnormalities.

On the basis of this information, we recommend that allergen immunotherapy be carefully continued during pregnancy in patients already receiving immunotherapy who appear to be deriving benefit therefrom and are not experiencing systemic reactions. For those women on maintenance therapy, a slightly lower maintenance dose may be considered so as to decrease the chance of a systemic reaction with coseasonal exposure. For women on an increasing antigen dosage schedule, either very conservative progression or no further increase in the dosage is recommended, again to minimize the risk of a systemic reaction. We do not believe that benefit/risk considerations favor beginning immunotherapy during pregnancy for most women since patients just beginning immuno-therapy (1) have an undefined propensity for systemic reaction, (2) may be more likely to experience systemic reactions with the frequent dosage increases that occur during initial treatment, (3) will derive an unpredictable amount of benefit, and (4) will experience a latency of immunotherapy effect.

Because skin testing with potent antigens may also be associated with systemic reactions, we recommend that skin tests be performed during pregnancy only if the results will have substantial therapeutic impact. In our experience, this is rarely the case since, even in patients not previously skin-tested, historical information will usually identify dust, mold, dander, or pollen sensitivities for which avoidance instructions may be empirically given. If allergen immunotherapy is not to be begun during pregnancy, knowledge of specific mold, mite, or pollen sensitivities can await postpartum testing. A few specific radioallergosorbent (RAST) tests may be ordered if confirmation of histori-cally relevant allergens seems necessary.

## Pharmacologic Management

Drugs are associated with two main types of adverse effect on the developing fetus: (1) they may act as teratogens when administered during weeks 3–10 of intrauterine life; and (2) although drugs prescribed after 10 weeks of intrauterine life should not be teratogenic, they may adversely affect the growth or function of normally formed tissues or organs. In addition, drugs taken by the lactating mother may enter breast milk to be ingested by the nursing infant. Thus the ideal pharmacologic therapy during pregnancy and lactation is no pharmacologic therapy, especially during the first trimester. However, a number of women with asthma require pharmacologic intervention to accomplish the goals of asthma therapy described above.

In evaluating a specific medication for use in treating asthma during pregnancy and lactation, one should take into account the results of both animal teratogenicity studies and human data on the use of that drug during pregnancy and lactation. Such information regarding medications commonly prescribed for asthmatic patients is summarized in Table 23-8 and may be found in more detail elsewhere.[2] One should also consider the efficacy and necessity of the medication, its route of administration (topical vs systemic), and how long the drug has been in clinical use. On the basis of all these considerations, a protocol for the pharmacologic management of asthma during pregnancy has been derived for use in the Kaiser Permanente Study of Asthma During Pregnancy (Table 23-9). This protocol is not meant to represent absolute or final recommendations, but rather working

**Table 23-8**

**Data on Use of Specific Medications During Pregnancy and Lactation**

| Drug | Animal Studies | Human Studies | Lactation |
|---|---|---|---|
| **Sympathomimetic bronchodilators** | | | |
| Epinephrine | Positive* in some species Vasoconstrictive effect of IV drug on monkey uteroplacental circulation | CPP †positive | NSIA‡ but would be destroyed in infants' GI tract |
| Ephedrine | Decreased monkey uterine blood flow following IV drug | CPP negative | NSIA |
| Isoproterenol | Positive in some species | CPP negative | NSIA but would be destroyed in infants' GI tract |
| Isoetharine | No data | No CPP data | NSIA |
| Metaproterenol | Positive in some species | No CPP data | NSIA |
| | | May inhibit term labor | |
| Albuteral | Positive in some species | Used to treat premature labor with maternal cardiac complications and certain neonatal complications reported | |
| Terbutaline | Negative* | Terbutaline may increase or preserve uterine blood flow | Amounts in milk probably small |
| **Other Asthma Medications** | | | |
| Theophylline | Positive in some species | CPP negative | Breast milk level 70% of serum level |
| | | Placental transfer documented | |
| | | May inhibit uterine contractions but less effectively than beta-2 sympathomimetics | Infant receives less than 10% of maternal dose |

**Table 23-8 Continued**

| Drug | Animal Studies | Human Studies | Lactation |
|---|---|---|---|
| Cromolyn | Negative | Use in 296 women not associated with increased complications | NSIA |
| Atropine | No data | CPP negative<br><br>Placental transfer with infant tachycardia documented | Amount in milk could inhibit lactation or cause atropine intoxication (although no good documentation) |
| Oral Corticosteroids | Positive in several species | CPP negative; see Table 23-9 | 0.07%–0.28% of maternal oral dose recovered per liter of milk |
| Beclomethasone | Negative (orally, inhalational) | No complications reported in 20 women in one series and no increase in congenital malformations reported in 45 pregnancies in another series | NSIA |
| Antihistamines | Hydroxyzine positive<br>Tripelennamine negative | CPP positive for brompheniramine, chlorpheniramine<br><br>CPP negative for tripelennamine<br><br>Diphenhydramine linked with cleft lip/palate in one series<br><br>No excess fetal abnormalities in 74 hydroxyzine-treated women compared to 34 controls | Amounts in milk probably small with no substantial adverse effect on milk supply or infant documented |

| Drug | | | NSIA |
|---|---|---|---|
| Oral Sympathomimetic Decongestants | Phenylephrine positive<br>Pseudephrine negative | CPP positive for phenylephrine, phenylpropanolimine<br>CPP negative for pseudephedrine | |
| Antibiotics<br>Penicillins | Negative | CPP negative | No adverse effects |
| Erythromycin | Positive in some species | CPP negative<br>Maternal toxicity with estolate but not other salt | No adverse effects |
| Cephalosporins | Negative | No CPP data | No adverse effects |
| Tetracycline | Positive in some species | Maternal hepatic toxicity<br>Can inhibit bone growth and cause hypoplasia and staining of teeth | Could theoretically cause mottling of teeth in infants, although may be bound by the calcium in milk and thus not be absorbed by the nursing infant |
| Sulfonamides | Positive in some species | Treatment in late pregnancy may cause fetal kernicterus | May cause hemolysis in G6PD-deficient infants<br>May cause jaundice or kernicterus in normal infants |

*For teratogenicity.
†Collaborative Perinatal Project study of congenital malformations associated with medication use during the first 4 months of pregnancy in 50,282 women (15).
‡No specific information available.
Adapted from Schatz M, Zeiger RS, Mellon M, et al: Asthma and allergic diseases during pregnancy: Management of the mother and prevention in the child in Middleton EL, Reed CE, Ellis EF (Eds): Allergy: Principles and Practice. St. Louis, Mosby, in press. (2)

Table 23-9
**A Suggested Protocol for Pharmologic Management of Asthma During Pregnancy**

I. Chronic
   A. Intermittent mild symptoms
      1. No medication
      2. Beta-2 Inhaled bronchodilator as needed
      3. Theophylline tablets as needed
   B. More continuous symptoms—regular theophylline
   C. Symptoms not controlled on above
      1. Mild-moderate symptoms: Consider ephedrine for short-term use
      2. Moderate symptoms
         a. Cromolyn (following beta-2 inhaled bronchodilator during initiation phase)
         b. Beclomethasone (following beta-2 inhaled bronchodilator during initation phase
      3. Moderate-severe continuous wheezing—clear with prednisone and consider (once clear)
         a. Theophylline
         b. Cromolyn
         c. Beclomethasone
         d. Alternate-day prednisone
         e. Daily prednisone
   D. Patients on medication prior to pregnancy
      1. Continue theophylline, cromolyn, beclomethasone, prednisone at lowest effective dose
      2. Try to substitute for or eliminate oral or high-dose inhalational beta-2 bronchodilators

II. Acute
   A. Oxygen
   B. Glucose-containing fluids
   C. Inhaled beta-2 sympathomimetics by mechanical nebulizer ($\leq$3 times, 20–30 min apart)
   D. For patients not responding to the above, IV aminophylline
      1. For patients not on oral theophylline, 5.6 mg/kg over 20–30 min
      2. For patients on oral theophylline, individual considerations (including time and amount of last oral theophylline dose, duration and amount of maintenance oral program, and known prior theophylline levels) will determine whether a half-loading dose (2.8 mg/kg over 20–30 min) should precede continuous IV administration
      3. If continuous aminophylline is indicated, administration by IVAC infusion pump at a dose of 0.4 mg/(kg h$^{-1}$) is initially recommended; Subsequent dose adjustments should be made on basis of frequent theophylline measurements
   E. Subcutaneous terbutaline once or twice should be considered for patients not tolerating inhaled bronchodilators and not responding to aminophylline or for patients in impending respiratory failure in spite of above therapy
   F. For patients responding slowly to the above within first few hours, or those initially severely ill, IV methylprednisolone should be given; usual dose 40–125 mg q 4–6 h

hypotheses that will be subject to confirmation or modification as additional data become available.

### Inhaled Bronchodilators

There is insufficient information on the use of inhaled sympathomimetics during pregnancy to allow one to identify the safest drug. The newer beta-2 agents may be preferred because of their longer duration of action and their increased bronchial selectivity. There is no specific information available on the use of inhaled bronchodilators during lactation, although one would not expect a substantial adverse effect.

### Theophylline

Theophylline is an effective and generally well-tolerated bronchodilator that has been used for over 40 years in this country without reported adverse effects during human pregnancy. In the Collaborative Perinatal Project (CPP) study[15] (see Table 23-8), nearly 200 women used theophylline or aminophylline during the first 4 months of pregnancy without any increased incidence of congenital malformations. Although placental transfer has been documented, adverse effects of placentally transferred theophylline in the newborn have been transient and rarely reported.[16] We thus consider chronic theophylline therapy the initial treatment of choice for most pregnant women with more continuous mild to moderate symptoms. We generally recommend sustained-release preparations, beginning with 375–500 mg/day in two to three divided doses and increasing as necessary and as tolerated with careful monitoring of the clinical response and the serum theophylline levels.

Preliminary pharmacokinetic data show that the volume of distribution for theophylline increases with pregnancy while the clearance remains constant.[17] This suggests that the milligram/kilogram basis for theophylline dosage may be unchanged during pregnancy but that the absolute requirement for theophylline might increase during the latter part of pregnancy. Thus theophylline levels should be repeated and dose adjustments considered in a previously controlled patient whose asthma becomes more troublesome in later pregnancy.

Although theophylline has been reported to inhibit uterine contractions,[18] this effect is substantially less than that of systemic beta-2 sympathomimetics. However, we have recently found that our multiparous asthmatic patients treated with theophylline during or within 24 hours of labor had significantly longer labors than control women or asthmatic patients not treated with bronchodilators (unpublished data). These multiparous theophylline-treated asthmatics did not experience increased complications of labor or delivery, and their infants exhibited no evidence of increased fetal distress, low Apgar scores or other abnormalities. Thus, since the occurrence of substantial asthma during labor would be more hazardous than this prolongation of labor, we recommend that theophylline be continued near term. However, one may wish to carefully taper theophylline dosage near term in well-controlled multiparous patients to ensure that these patients are receiving the lowest dose of theophylline that will control their asthma when labor occurs.

Theophylline passes into breast milk, where its concentration is about 70% of the maternal serum level.[19] However, it is estimated that the infant receives less than 10% of the maternal dose. Although nursing infants should be monitored for the pharmacologic actions of theophylline, irritability may thus be the most serious (and relatively infrequent) adverse effect encountered in this setting.

### Oral Beta Sympathomimetics

Ephedrine is the oldest oral bronchodilator drug in clinical use today, and 373 women in the CPP study[15] (see Table 23-8) used ephedrine during the first 4 months of pregnancy without any increased occurrence of congenital malformations. However, because tachyphylaxis has been reported with the chronic use of ephedrine, we do not consider it to be a first-line medication for chronic bronchodilator therapy during pregnancy. Ephedrine may be useful, though, for short-term use in a patient already on a maximal dose of theophylline for a mild to moderate exacerbation such as may be associated with an upper respiratory infection.

There are no first trimester human data on metaproterenol, terbutaline, or albuterol, but animal studies have been positive for metaproterenol and albuterol. In addition, all three of these beta-2 agents have been shown to have enough inhibitory effect on the uterus that they have been used clinically to suppress premature labor. When they are used in this setting, certain maternal and neonatal complications have been reported. For all these reasons, we try to avoid systemic beta-2 sympathomimetics during pregnancy, if possible. Although full-dose regular inhalational therapy provides less of a systemic dose, the possibility of adverse effects from this smaller but not necessarily insignificant dose cannot be excluded on the basis of the available data. Consequently, long-term, high-dose inhalational sympathomimetic therapy during pregnancy cannot be recommended at this time.

For patients controlled on oral beta-2 sympathomimetics prior to pregnancy, we recommend a trial of conversion to oral theophylline if the patient is or plans to become pregnant. For patients in whom an oral beta sympathomimetic appears to be an essential part of the therapeutic program, one may consider switching to ephedrine. However, since ephedrine may be neither as effective nor as well-tolerated as the new oral beta-2 sympathomimetics, an occasional patient may have to remain on one of these agents during pregnancy. In such a patient, it may still be possible to taper or discontinue this medication in the few weeks prior to term, when asthma improves in most patients, and when the use of this medication may be most problematic.

Little terbutaline is secreted in the breast milk, and apparently the amount is not harmful to the nursing infant. There is no specific information available on the use of the other oral sympathomimetics during lactation.

### Cromolyn and Beclomethasone

Animal teratogenicity studies with cromolyn have been negative, and Wilson[20] has recently reported on 296 women who used cromolyn during their entire pregnancy with no apparent increase in complications. Morrow-Brown and Storey[21] described the use of beclomethasone in 20 pregnant women with no complications, and, more recently, Greenberger and Patterson[22] have reported on the use of beclomethasone during 45 pregnancies with no increased prevalence of congenital malformations. We thus recommend cromolyn or beclomethasone for patients chronically uncontrolled on full-dose oral theophylline. We would generally recommend that cromolyn be considered first. Patients requiring cromolyn or beclomethasone prior to pregnancy should continue the medication during pregnancy, unless there appears to be such a change in clinical course that it may no longer be required. Since cromolyn and beclomethasone are relatively new drugs and do not have an established safety record during pregnancy, they should be used only with the patient's informed consent. Although there is no specific information available on the use of these medications during lactation, one would not expect significant amounts of either drug to appear in breast milk.

### Systemic Corticosteroids

Although animal studies have suggested adverse effects of systemic corticosteroids on the developing fetus, most of the human data have not confirmed a substantial adverse effect. Table 23-10 describes the outcome in 255 asthmatic women reported in the literature who were treated with corticosteroids during pregnancy.

Table 23-10
Use of Corticosteroids During Pregnancy in Asthmatic Patients

| Study | Number of Pregnancies > 20 Weeks | Perinatal Deaths, % | Preterm Infants, % | Congenital Malformations, % |
|---|---|---|---|---|
| Total | 255 | 2.9 | 15.3 | Total: 3.3 Cleft Palate/lip 1.2 Spina bifida 0.8 |
| Control | — | 1.5–3.2 | 5–18 | Total: 2–3 Cleft palate/lip 0.15 Spina bifida 0.065 |
| Gordon et al. (1) | 277 | 5.9 | 14.4 | — |
| Walsh and Grant (24) | 17 | 17.6 | — | Total: 5.9 |
| Warrell and Taylor (23) | 18 | 16.7 | 20.0 | Total: 0.0 |

Adapted from Schatz M, Zeiger RS, Mellon M, et al: Asthma and allergic diseases during pregnancy: Management of the mother and prevention in the child: In Middleton EL, Reed CE, Ellis EF (Eds): Allergy: Principles and Practice. St. Louis, Mosby, in press.[2]

Also shown in Table 23-10 are the data from the studies by Gordon et al.[1] in asthmatic patients, treatment unspecified, as well as the results of two series that showed an inordinately high incidence of complications in corticosteroid-treated asthmatics.[23,24] The overall series of 255 patients demonstrates no increased incidence of perinatal deaths, preterm births, or total congenital malformations as well as no increased rate of abortions or pregnancy complications compared to general population figures. The reasons for the frequency of adverse consequences in the studies by Warrell and Taylor[23] and that of Walsh and Grant[24] are not immediately apparent. However, the perinatal mortality in the accumulated series is less than half that occurring in the women with gestational asthma in the large study by Gordon et al.[1] Moreover, a stillbirth associated with status asthmaticus during labor occurred in one of the "control" asthmatics not treated with corticosteroids in the study by Warrell and Taylor.[23] Although there did appear to be an increased incidence of cleft lip, cleft palate, and spina bifida in the steroid-treated women compared to general population figures, these data are difficult to interpret in this relatively small series of patients who were probably treated with multiple medications. From the overall data, we conclude that corticosteroids should be used when indicated for the management of moderate to severe asthma during pregnancy. For patients who are corticosteroid-dependent prior to pregnancy, corticosteroids should be continued at the lowest dose that will achieve control (which may change during pregnancy if the course of asthma changes).

Prednisone and prednisolone are commonly used for the treatment of asthma in the nongravid state and appear to be good choices for use during pregnancy based on maternal–fetal gradient data. At this time the information available regarding the pharmacokinetics of corticosteroids administered during pregnancy is insufficient for recommendation of any different dosing schedules in the gravid and the nongravid state.

Data on the use of oral prednisone during lactation suggest that 0.07%–0.28% of the maternal dose is recovered per liter of milk.[25,26] Thus the use of corticosteroids at usual oral doses in the lactating mother appears to be no substantial threat to the infant.

*Parenteral Sympathomimetics*

Epinephrine has been associated with increased congenital malformations in one animal study and in the CPP study.[15] In addition, IV epinephrine has been shown to have vasoconstrictive effects on the uteroplacental circulation of monkeys. As discussed earlier, there are no first-trimester human teratogenicity data for terbutaline, but terbutaline may inhibit labor at term. For these reasons, our protocol for the treatment of acute asthma during pregnancy tries to minimize the use of parenteral sympathomimetics. In certain patients with severe acute asthma not responding to other therapy, however, it appears that the benefits of parenteral sympathomimetics still may outweigh the potential risks. Although terbutaline is a newer drug, animal teratogenicity studies have been negative, and it has been shown to preserve or increase uterine blood flow in humans. When parenteral sympathomimetics are required during pregnancy, therefore, terbutaline may be a better choice than epinephrine.

*Other Medications*

Antihistamines, sympathomimetic decongestants, and antibiotics may be necessary for the treatment of associated rhinitis or complicating respiratory infections during pregnancy. On the basis of the available data, tripelennamine appears to be the antihistamine, and pseudephedrine the decongestant, of choice during pregnancy. Penicillins, cephalosporins, and erythromycin (other than the estolate salt) appear safe during pregnancy and lactation, whereas tetracycline is contraindicated and sulfonamides should be avoided during late pregnancy and lactation.

Iodides (e.g., SSKI [Upsher-Smith Laboratories, Inc, Minneapolis, MN], Quadrinal [Knoll Pharmaceutical Company, Whippany, NJ]) are contraindicated during pregnancy and lactation because of their potential for producing life-threatening fetal goiter. Phenobarbital has been associated with congenital malformations in two human series, and thus combination bronchodilators containing phenobarbitol should be avoided during pregnancy. Prostaglandins used to induce labor have been associated with bronchoconstriction and should be avoided if possible in patients with asthma.

## Management During Labor

Obstetric management during labor of the controlled asthmatic woman is identical to the management of the nonasthmatic patient. When general anesthesia is necessary, halogenated agents are desirable since they possess broncholytic activities. Although exacerbations of asthma during labor are uncommon, we recommend that patients on oral theophylline or inhaled cromolyn or beclomethasone continue this therapy through labor. As noted above, patients on theophylline should be treated with the lowest effective dose. Patients on oral theophylline who require surgical intervention may receive IV aminophylline instead.

Steroid-dependent asthmatics should receive supplemental steroids for the stress of labor, delivery, and the puerperium. The following regimen has been recommended:[3] 100 mg of hydrocortisone intramuscularly (IM) every 8 hours for 24 hours or until the absence of puerperal complications is established. Adrenal insufficiency has only rarely been reported in infants of mothers receiving corticosteroids during pregnancy. Consequently, although such infants should be carefully observed for any evidence of adrenal hypofunction, prophylactic treatment is not warranted.

# REFERENCES

1. Gordon M, Niswander KR, Berendes H, et al: Fetal morbidity following potentially anoxigenic obstetric conditions. Am J Ob Gyn 106:421–429, 1970

2. Schatz M, Zeiger RS, Mellon M, et al: In Middleton EL, Reed CE, Ellis EF (Eds): Allergy: Principles and Practice, St. Louis, Mosby, in press

3. Turner ES, Greenberger PA, Patterson R: Management of the pregnant asthmatic patient. Ann Int Med 6:905–918, 1980

4. Weinstein AM, Dubin BD, Posleski WK, et al: Asthma and pregnancy. JAMA 241:1161–1165, 1979

5. Jaffe RB: In Yen SC, Jaffe RB (Eds): Reproductive Endocrinology: Physiology, Pathophysiology, and Clinical Management, 1978, Philadelphia, Saunders, pp 521–536

6. Weinberger SE, Weiss ST, Cohen WR, et al: Pregnancy and the lung. Am Rev Respir Dis 121:559–581, 1980

7. Beer AE, Billingham RE: The Immunology of Mammalian Reproduction, Englewood Cliffs, NJ, Prentice-Hall, 1976

8. Sorri M, Hartikainen-Sorri AL, Karja J: Rhinitis during pregnancy. Rhinology 18:83–86, 1980

9. Gluck JC, Gluck PA: The effects of pregnancy on asthma: A prospective study. Ann Allergy 37:164–168, 1976

10. Bahna SL, Bjerkedal T: The course and outcome of pregnancy in women with bronchial asthma. Acta Allergol 27:397–406, 1972

11. Williams DA: Asthma and pregnancy. Acta Allergol (Kbh) 22:311–323, 1967

12. Brown WA: Psychological Care During Pregnancy and the Postpartum Period, New York, Raven Press, 1979

13. Francis N: Abortion after grass pollen injection. J Allergy 12:559–563, 1941

14. Metzger WI, Turner E, Patterson R: The safety of immunotherapy during pregnancy. J Allergy Clin Immunol 61:268–272, 1978

15. Heinonen OD, Slone D, Shapiro S: Birth defects and drugs in pregnancy, Littleton, MA, PSG Publishing Co., 1977

16. Arwood LL, Dasta JF, Friedman C: Placental transfer of theophylline: Two case reports. Pediatrics 63:844–846, 1979

17. Sutton PL, Koup JR, Rose JQ, et al: The pharmacokinetics of theophylline in pregnancy. J Allergy Clin Immunol 61:174 (abstr), 1978

18. Lipshitz J: Uterine and cardiovascular effects of aminophylline. Am J Ob Gyn 131:716–718, 1978

19. Stec GP, Greenberger P, Ruo TI, et al: Kinetics of theophylline transfer to breast milk. Clin Pharm Ther 28:404–408, 1980

20. Wilson J: Utilisation du cromoglycate du sodium au cours de la grossesse. Acta Ther 8 (Suppl):45–51, 1982

21. Morrow-Brown H, Story G: Beclomethason dipropionate aerosol in long-term treatment of perennial and seasonal asthma in children and adults: a report of five and one-half years experience in 600 asthmatic patients. Br J Clin Pharm 4:2595–2675, 1977

22. Greenberger PA, Patterson R: Beclomethason dipropionate for severe asthma during pregnancy. Ann Int Med 98:478–480, 1983

23. Warrell DW, Taylor R: Outcome for the foetus of mothers receiving prednisolone during pregnancy. Lancet 1:117–118, 1968

24. Walsh SD, Grant WB: Corticosteroids in treatment of chronic asthma. Br Med J 2:796–802, 1966

25. Berlin CM: In Yaffe SJ (Ed): Pediatric Pharmacology, New York, Grune & Stratton, 1980, pp 137–147

26. McKenzie SA, Selley JA, Agnar JE: Secretion of prednisolone into breast milk. Arch Dis Childh 50:894–896, 1975

# 24

JORDAN FINK

## Occupational Asthma

Ramazzini[1] was the first to recognize that the patient's occupation must be considered when evaluating an illness. He described attacks of shortness of breath following inhalation of occupational environmental dusts in sifters and millers of grain.

Since Ramazzini's time, many types of occupational dust have been incriminated in respiratory disease. Vegetable dusts and metal salts were initially recognized as causative agents in this century, and more recently the manufacture of plastics has introduced a number of highly reactive chemicals into the work environment that have been associated with the development of asthma and other respiratory illnesses. The occupational history may be of great diagnostic importance. It is essential that the physician pay attention to the workplace and occupational exposures in evaluating an asthmatic patient, even when it appears that the asthma is caused mainly by pollens, molds, house dust, or animal danders.

### PREVALENCE

The prevalence of asthma has been estimated at 3% of the population, and of that number anywhere from 2% to 15% have been considered occupational in origin. Thus there may be close to one million individuals with occupational asthma in this country.[2] These individuals must represent a significant fraction of the 500,000 cases of occupational disease estimated by the U.S. Department of Labor to occur each year.

The prevalence of asthma in the workplace varies widely with occupation. In a study of a platinum refining industry, over 50% of workers exposed to platinum salts developed respiratory symptoms, and after 5 years of contact, nearly all workers had symptoms.[3] In the baking industry, 10%–20% of individuals exposed to flour developed symptoms. Another important industry in which occupational asthma is prevalent is pharmaceutical manufacturing. Antibiotics such as penicillin may be contacted by inhalation in the environment of manufacturing plants, and sensitization of workers may result.[3] It has become apparent that with increasing exposure to occupational chemicals and other materials, cases of occupational asthma will be on the increase.

### PREDISPOSING FACTORS

Atopy, or the tendency to develop IgE-antibody-mediated disease, is a predisposing factor in some occupational situations. Atopic individuals appear more likely to develop IgE-antibody-mediated asthma as a result of the inhalation of enzymes of *Bacillus subtilis*

**213**

used in the manufacture of washing powders.[4] Asthma in wood workers, however, occurs mainly in nonatopic individuals. When the intensity and duration of exposure is sufficient, asthma may perhaps result in the ordinarily nonatopic individual. Also, it is likely that the most sensitive individuals quickly develop symptoms and quit their jobs leaving behind a less susceptible population who develop symptoms more gradually. On the other hand, if the degree of exposure is not great, or if IgE-antibody-mediated mechanisms are not involved in the production of the symptoms, atopy may not be important.

## TYPES OF ASTHMA

Occupational asthma may occur as a result of several mechanisms. Antigen inhalation may sensitize through the production of IgE antibodies. Bronchospasm may be induced by the inhalation of irritative substances or materials that release histamine or other mediators. Several features of occupational asthma point to mediation by IgE antibody mechanisms. Attacks occurring after a period of sensitization suggest IgE mechanisms, whereas those appearing at the first exposure would be indicative of an irritant effect. The attack rate of allergic occupational respiratory disease is low, with only a small proportion of workers affected. The reaction becomes more severe with increased duration of exposure and may ultimately become persistent asthma. With more severe asthma, systemic symptoms such as chills, mild fever, malaise, and joint aches may occur.

Other diagnostic aids to occupational asthma include the demonstration of an immediate wheal-and-flare skin reaction to antigens found in the patient's occupational environment. Coffee bean handlers, flour workers, and platinum workers typically develop skin reactions in association with asthma.[3]

Occupational asthma in which no clear-cut immunologic mechanism can be detected is also common (Table 24-1). Asthma associated with toluene diisocyanate (TDI) in the plastics industry is well recognized. Approximately 15% of individuals with TDI-induced asthma have IgE antibodies to a TDI-protein conjugate. A small number of workers have demonstrable cellular immune responses detected by lymphokine generation and blastogenesis with appropriate antigen.[5] The majority of individuals sensitized, however, have no demonstrable immune response; some may have asthma as a result of enhancement of beta-adrenergic blockade by TDI. The degree of sensitization may be extreme; as little as 0.002 ppm may induce a respiratory response, whereas 0.01–0.02 ppm has been advocated as a safe industrial level.[6]

The heating of polyvinyl chloride during the hot-wire cutting of meat wrapping material has been associated with asthma. The symptoms have been thought to be related to inhalation of pyrolisis products of the heated soft wrap film, although recently inhalation of fumes from thermoactivated label glue have also been associated with respiratory distress. The problem has disappeared with the use of a cool-wire cutting process and the complete enclosure of the wrapping and labeling procedures.

Other mechanisms resulting in occupational asthma include reflex bronchoconstriction induced by cold air and by low concentrations of sulfur dioxide, fluorocarbons, and various inert dusts. Inflammation resulting in bronchoconstriction may be due to inhalation of toxic gases such as ammonia, sulfur dioxide, halogen fumes, acids, and chemical solvents.[7] Byssinosis, seen in the cotton textile industry, is most commonly found amongst the workers who are exposed to the initial processing stages, especially with cotton of low-quality containing bract, the vegetable fiber that adheres to the cotton boll. It

Table 24-1
**Agents Associated with Occupational Asthma**

| Agent | Occupation |
| --- | --- |
| IgE-Antibody-Mediated | |
| Coffee and castor beans | Dock workers, millers |
| Pancreatic extracts | Food workers |
| Papain | Food workers |
| Enzymes from *B. subtilis* | Detergent workers |
| Platinum salts | Refiners, chemists |
| Phenylglycine acid chloride | Pharmaceutical workers |
| Flour | Bakers |
| Gum acacia | Printers |
| Phthalic anhydride | Plastics industry |
| Trimelitic anhydride | Plastics industry |
| Toluene diisocyanate (15% of workers) | Plastics industry |
| Non-IgE-Antibody-Mediated | |
| Toluene diisocyanate (15% of workers) | Plastics industry |
| Wood dusts | Wood workers |
| Pyrolisis products of plastic wrap | Meat wrappers |
| Soldering flux | Electrical workers |
| Cotton | Ginners, millers |

has been shown that extracts from cotton bract can release histamine from chopped human lung tissue.[8] It is likely that this direct release of mediator induces the bronchospasm associated with this occupation.

## BRONCHIAL REACTIONS

Bronchial provocation carried out in the laboratory under controlled conditions has demonstrated a number of patterns of response that reproduce the symptoms that follow work exposure to sensitizing antigens. Analysis of the symptoms associated with exposure at work may provide important clues as to the etiology of the patient's disorder.

*Immediate* asthma occurs within minutes of exposure to the offending antigen, is maximum at 20–30 minutes, and lasts for up to 2 hours. It is readily reversible with bronchodilators and is prevented by prior administration of sodium cromolyn but not by corticosteroids. It is typically induced by IgE antibody–antigen interaction with mediator release from mast cells. *Late-onset* asthma begins one to several hours after inhalation of the offending agent, has a gradual onset, is progressive, and is often more severe than immediate asthma. The bronchospasm may be predominantly in the small airways and may last for up to 36 hours. Symptoms are typically shortness of breath rather than wheezing. The symptoms and pulmonary function abnormalities respond poorly to bronchodilators but well to corticosteroids; they may also be prevented by prior administration of corticosteroids.[9] *Dual* asthma begins as an immediate response with typical pulmonary function change in the $FEV_1$ that returns to normal within 2 hours. A second phase of the asthmatic response begins several hours later and is of the late-onset asthma type. *Repetitive* asthma beings as a late-onset type, only to recur periodically for several days after a single initial exposure. The mechanisms inducing the nonimmediate forms of asthma are not known, although there is some evidence that the delayed-onset types may be related to late release of mediators or release of mediators with late action.[3]

## DIAGNOSIS

### History and Physical Examination

A detailed description of the workers' symptoms is of great importance in the diagnosis of occupational asthma. If the symptoms occur within minutes of contact with a specific agent and on cessation of exposure, there is probably a cause and effect relationship between the environment and the symptoms. In delayed-onset asthma, symptoms begin after the exposure, for example, when the patient is at home. Shortness of breath and cough rather than wheeze may predominate. With continued exposure the latent period often decreases and the duration of the symptoms increases. The patient then has continuous asthma and appears to have chronic lung disease. A careful history is necessary to relate such symptoms to the workplace.

Physical examination features vary with the patient's status and pulmonary function. There may be overt wheezing and rhonchi or just depressed breath sounds depending on the type and duration of asthma. Clearing may be rapid or gradual with avoidance or with appropriate medication.

### Laboratory Tests

Skin testing with a battery of common inhalant antigens can be useful in determining whether the patient is atopic. It can also be useful in evaluating the immediate skin reactivity of materials to which the patient has been exposed. In order to use low-molecular-weight chemicals as skin test reagents, conjugates to proteins such as human serum albumin may be necessary.

Radioallergosorbent (RAST) tests have been useful in demonstrating IgE antibodies to low-molecular-weight chemicals. Inhalation challenge tests with toluene diisocyanate and trimelitic anhydride have been helpful in evaluating occupational exposures and sensitization of workers.

### Pulmonary Function Tests

Spirometry, with measurements of one second forced expiratory volume ($FEV_1$), forced vital capacity (FVC), and midexpiratory flow ($FEF_{25-75}$) are often adequate for evaluation of workers. Significant changes occurring from pre- to postwork shift on workdays with no changes at similar times on nonworkdays may indicate the presence of a bronchial reactant in the work environment.

Inhalation challenge testing using increasing concentrations of methacholine may induce a significant (greater than 20%) change in $FEV_1$ from baseline. This change indicates hyperactive airways and is helpful in making a diagnosis of asthma. Bronchial hyperactivity is a usual finding in occupational asthma.

## Bronchial Challenge

The technique of bronchial challenge provides a method for reproducing the patient's pulmonary response to an occupational agent suspected of causing the symptoms and can also be of value in identifying the specific agent to which the worker is sensitive. Once the agent is identified, it can more readily be avoided.

The technique is aimed at reproducing the patient's work environment in the laboratory. However, at times it may be more practical to evaluate the patient at the place of work. It is best to use the suspected agent in the form in which it is encountered by the worker rather than in an adulterated form. For example, fine powders, dusts, and fumes from volatile substances may be utilized in the challenge tests. Pulmonary function tests are carried out before and at intervals after challenge and are compared to controls. Significant changes and reproduction of one of the patterns of response described earlier will pinpoint the offending agents and allow a diagnosis.

## THERAPY

Prevention of occupational asthma is of prime importance and environmental control is the means for prevention once causative agents have been identified. The work environment should be monitored for dusts or chemicals known to be potent inducers of asthma. Areas where they are detected should be appropriately ventilated, and workers in those areas should be protected with masks.

Sensitive workers may be moved to areas remote from exposure to an offending agent. If this is not practicable, a change of employment may be necessary.

Drugs may effectively control the symptoms but avoidance is more desirable. Cromolyn sodium may be effective in blocking the asthmatic response. In some cases theophylline preparations or beta-agonists may be of value. If the symptoms are severe enough to require corticosteroid treatment, a change of environment is preferable to the long-term use of these agents.

## REFERENCES

1.  Ramazzini B: DeMorbis Artificum Diatriba (Wright WC, transl). Chicago, University of Chicago Press, 1940 (original publication in 1713)
2.  Introna F: L'asma bronchale allergica come malattia professionale. Minerva Medicoleg 86:176–184, 1966
3.  Pepys J, Davies RJ: Occupational asthma. In Middleton E, Reed CE, Ellis EF (Eds): Allergy, Principles and Practice, St. Louis, Mosby, 1978, pp 812–842
4.  Slavin RG, Lewis CR: Sensitivity to enzyme additives in laundry detergent workers. J Allergy Clin Immunol 48:262–266, 1971
5.  Gallagher JS, Tse CS, Brooks SM, et al: Diverse profiles if immunoreactivity in toluene diisocyanate asthma. J Occup Med 23: 610–616, 1981
6.  Karr RM, Davies, RJ, Butcher BT, et al: Occupational asthma. J Allergy Clin Immunol 61:54–65, 1978
7.  Bernstein IL: Occupational asthma. Clin Chest Med 2:255–272, 1981
8.  Bouhys A, Lindell SE: Release of histamine by cotton dust extracts from human lung tissue in-vitro. Experentia 17:211–218

9.  Pepys J: Hypersensitivity disease of the lungs due to fungi and other organic dusts. In Monographs in Allergy, Basel, S. Karger, 1969

## SUGGESTED READINGS

Lutsky I, Toshner D: A review of allergic respiratory disease in laboratory animal workers. Lab Animal Sci 28:751–756, 1978

## 25

ROBERT B. SARNOFF

# Management of the Bronchospastic Patient Through a Major Surgical Procedure

Asthmatic patients must be carefully prepared for major surgical operations, especially those involving the chest and abdomen. Although this is well recognized, it is all too common for the chest specialist to be asked to see a patient with a prior history of asthma who exhibits tachypnea, wheeze, and poor air movement. The bronchospastic patient who escapes these early postoperative troubles may still experience the later complications of atelectasis and pneumonia, which add to discomfort and prolong the hospital stay. This chapter reviews the effect of a surgical procedure on lung mechanics and pulmonary function and outlines a practical approach to the pre- and postoperative care of the bronchospastic patient.

## PATHOPHYSIOLOGIC CHANGES AFTER A MAJOR SURGICAL OPERATION

After a surgical operation there are characteristic changes in the lung volumes, the pattern of ventilation, gas exchange, and pulmonary defense mechanisms. These are seen in normal individuals and occur to an exaggerated degree in the bronchospastic patient. They are more severe when there has been immobilization, heavy use of pain medications, or prolonged anesthesia. Typically the vital capacity and the expiratory reserve volume (difference between the functional residual capacity and the residual volume) are diminished, probably because of pain and splinting of the chest and upper abdominal wall. The vital capacity is reduced by as much as 75% after thoractomy and by 60% after upper abdominal procedures.[1]

Disruption of the bony thorax, interference with the muscles of the chest wall, and, in the case of upper abdominal surgery, compromise of diaphragmatic function all contribute to the reduced vital capacity (VC). The greatest changes in vital capacity are noted in thoracic and upper abdominal procedures, with lesser reductions after lower abdominal operations (55% reduction in VC after upper abdominal surgery versus 40% reduction in VC in lower abdominal surgery). There are only minimal changes after nonthoracic and nonabdominal operations.[2,3] Changes in the functional residual capacity (FRC) after surgical procedures have especially important effects on gas exchange. The FRC is the volume of gas remaining in the lungs at the end of a normal expiration, and it has an important relationship to the closing capacity. The expiratory reserve volume (difference between the FRC and the residual volume) is reported to drop approximately 33% following all types of abdominal surgery.[3] This could cause the end tidal volume to fall below the closing capacity (the lung volume where the small airways collapse), thus encouraging absorption atelectasis with consequent hypoxemia due to venous admixture. The greater the reduction in the FRC and expiratory reserve volume, the greater the tendency to small airways closure, hypoxemia, and atelectasis. Therefore, these complications are especially common in operations on the chest and upper abdomen.

The pattern of ventilation is altered after a surgical operation. There is a 20% reduction in tidal volume within 24 hours after either abdominal or thoracic procedures, and the respiratory rate increases concurrently.[4] Although the minute ventilation changes relatively little, the work of breathing and the oxygen consumption may escalate considerably, leading to respiratory muscle fatigue and sometimes respiratory failure. The frequency of sighing is often decreased, which further encourages collapse of basal alveoli, reduced lung compliance, and increased work of breathing.[5] The decreased lung volumes, altered pattern of ventilation, and reduced sighing frequency all contribute to an insidious progression of alveolar collapse, retention of secretions, venous admixture, and hypoxemia. Finally, there is impairment of cough due to a combination of factors including pain, and analgesic medications. In the bronchospastic patient the decreased maximal inspiratory lung volume and the reduced maximal expiratory flow further interfere with the effectiveness of cough.

## Clinical Significance of These Pathophysiologic Changes

In the first few days after a surgical procedure these pathophysiologic changes may express themselves as pneumonia or atelectasis. A vicious cycle begins of chest wall and abdominal pain leading to reduced cough and sighing frequency. The lung volumes and lung compliance progressively decline, with increasing collapse of basal alveoli and worsening hypoxemia. Initial microatelectasis progresses to frank atelectasis, further impairing already abnormal ventilation–perfusion relationships. The collapsed regions are especially susceptible to bacterial infection, and pneumonia may be superimposed on atelectasis.

Atelectasis and pneumonia after a surgical procedure are hazards in all patients but are especially likely to occur in the asthmatic. If the bronchospastic patient can be identified prior to an operation and is appropriately treated both before and after the operation, the risk of postoperative complications can be significantly reduced. In 1962 Stein et al.[6] showed that the incidence of postoperative pulmonary complications in patients with abnormal pulmonary function was 70% as compared to only 34% in patients with normal preoperative spirometry.[6] Age, smoking, and obesity are other important risk factors. Boushy et al.[7] reported that postoperative complication rates were higher in patients above 60 years of age with an $FEV_1$ of less than 2 liters. As long ago as 1946, Dripps and Deming[8] showed that a "stir-up" program continued through pre- and postoperative periods reduced the incidence of atelectasis and pneumonia in over 1000 patients receiving a general anesthetic from 11% to 4%. In 1954, Thoren[9] emphasized the efficacy of chest physical therapy in reducing postoperative complications and showed that to achieve good compliance, the patient had to be carefully instructed before the operation. Stein,[10] who had earlier shown that the patient with obstructive lung disease was at increased risk of postoperative complications, showed reduced complication rates in high-risk patients who had preoperative and postoperative therapy directed at their lung disease.

## MANAGEMENT OF THE BRONCHOSPASTIC PATIENT THROUGH A MAJOR OPERATION

The usual careful history and physical examination should be supplemented by a chest x-ray and spirometry. If the spirogram shows more than mild bronchial obstruction, arterial blood gas analysis should also be performed. Even in the patient with a remote history of bronchospasm, a spirogram is advisable to assess the severity of flow obstruction and bronchodilator responsiveness.

If the physical examination and the spirometry are normal, it should be sufficient to observe the patient carefully after the operation for signs of bronchospasm. If bronchospasm does become a problem, it should be treated promptly and aggressively in the usual manner with intravenous (IV) aminophylline, inhaled sympathomimetics, and, if the bronchospasm is severe, with glucocorticoid injections. Patients with mild to moderate bronchospasm ($FEV_1$ 50%–70% of predicted levels) on no specific therapy at the time of initial evaluation should be given oral theophylline and inhaled sympathomimetics several days prior to operation. It is a matter of judgment whether to augment this program with a burst of prednisone, but, in general, the risks of a few days of a systemic corticosteroid will be far outweighed by the potential benefits. If there is evidence of bronchial hypersecretion and active infection, the patient should be admitted 2–3 days before the operation for respiratory therapy treatments aimed at mobilizing secretions and maintaining bronchodilatation (chest physical therapy and sympathomimetic aerosol treatment). If the operation is elective and if it appears that the patient would benefit from a few more days of preparation, the physician should not hesitate to recommend that the procedure be delayed.

Patients with moderate to severe bronchial obstruction should be started on IV methylprednisolone and aminophylline 12–24 hours before their surgery. Intravenous treatment should be initiated several days before the operation in patients with unstable bronchospasm who are considered at high risk of an acute asthmatic attack. Adequate corticosteroid therapy is especially important in patients currently receiving a steroid agent and in patients with a history of steroid dependence and severe bronchospastic disease.

Patients should be urged to discontinue smoking at least a few days before the operation and should be carefully instructed in the techniques of deep breathing and coughing. If incentive spirometry is used, the patient should be familiarized with the equipment before the operation.

## REFERENCES

1. Shapiro BA, Harrison RA, Trout CA: Acute restrictive disease. In Clinical Application of Respiratory Care, Chicago, Yearbook Medical, 1975
2. Beecher HK: Effect of laparotomy on lung volume. Demonstration of a new type of pulmonary collapse. J Clin Invest 12:651, 1933
3. Anscombe AR, Buxton RStJ: Effect of abdominal operations on total lung capacity and its subdivisions. Br Med J 2:84, 1958

4.  Beecher HK: The measured effect of laparotomy on the respiration. J Clin Invest 12:639, 1933

5.  Egbert LD, Bendixin HH: Atelectasis in the surgical patient. Recent conceptual advances. Progr Surg 5:1, 1966

6.  Stein M, Koota GM, Simon M, et al: Pulmonary evaluation of surgical patients. JAMA 181:765, 1962

7.  Boushy SF, Billeg DM, North LB, et al: Clinical course related to preoperative and postoperative pulmonary function on patients with bronchogenic carcinoma. Chest 59:383, 1971

8.  Dripps RD, Deming MVN: Postoperative atelectasis and pneumonia. Diagnosis etiology, and management based upon 1240 cases of upper abdominal surgery. Ann Surg 124:94, 1946

9.  Thoren L: Postoperative pulmonary complications. Observations on their prevention by means of physical therapy. Acta Chir Scand 107:193, 1954

10. Stein M, Cassara EL: Preoperative pulmonary evaluation and therapy for surgical patients. JAMA 211:787, 1970

# Hospital Management of the Severe Asthmatic in Relapse

One of the major goals in treating the severe asthmatic is to avoid hospitalization. The most effective means of accomplishing this is to educate patients about their diseases so that they will recognize and seek treatment for exacerbations before they become severe. The need for hospitalization can be reduced in patients with chronic obstructive lung disease after they have attended a multidisciplinary pulmonary rehabilitation program.[1,2] Some patients with severe chronic asthma should be considered for such programs. This education process may be life-saving. One study from England showed that 37% of 53 asthma deaths occurred outside the hospital without any contact with a physician.[3]

## THE DECISION TO HOSPITALIZE

Even with excellent physician–patient communication and a well-informed patient, the management of a severe exacerbation may require hospitalization. In the hospital one can provide the several days of close monitoring necessary to manage severe bronchospasm and, when appropriate, parenteral medications, intensive respiratory therapy, and mechanical ventilation.

The asthmatic arriving by ambulance in profound distress and requiring vigorous emergency care, if not resuscitation, obviously must be admitted. Minor exacerbations can generally be handled in the physician's office or the emergency room. A period of observation and some clinical judgment are needed before a decision is made whether to admit a patient with a moderately severe asthmatic relapse. The patient probably should be hospitalized if cough, chest tightness, and dyspnea persist after several days of a maximal program of theophylline, sympathomimetic, and corticosteroid medications in therapeutic doses. An important clue to a failing outpatient program is when a patient has had several emergency room or office visits within recent weeks for an exacerbation that has persisted. The patient may have improved after each visit, only to worsen within a few days. Lack of sleep due to asthmatic symptoms is another important feature of the history that should suggest the need for hospital care.

Although the history is helpful, objective information is usually needed to assess the severity of an exacerbation of asthma. Spirometry is the most valuable test and the $FEV_1$ the most reliable number for grading the degree of bronchial obstruction. Important points to note in the physical examination include the respiratory rate, the pulse rate, the presence of paradoxical pulse, and the recruitment of accessory respiratory muscles. The arterial blood gas is important in identifying evidence of respiratory failure, but a patient with normal blood gases can still be in urgent need of hospital care. This point is discussed in further detail later.

## ACCURACY OF THE DIAGNOSIS

The history and physical findings are usually characteristic enough to lead the physician rapidly to a correct diagnosis, and spirometry provides objective confirmation. However, for a severe asthmatic it is worth considering a few other conditions that may masquerade as asthma or coexist with it. These include upper airway obstruction, chronic obstructive airways disease, aspiration, thromboembolism, pulmonary venous hypertension, and hyperventilation syndrome.

### Upper Airway Obstruction

Obstruction of the upper airways at any level from the nasopharynx to the trachea can masquerade as asthma, even to the extent of partial response to bronchodilator therapy. Patients who have been intubated in the past may develop granulation tissue or fibrous stenosis of the larnyx or trachea. Signs suggesting upper airways obstruction include inspiratory stridor and when the obstruction is severe, a characteristic abnormal pattern on the spirogram. The spirometric features are best illustrated on a flow volume loop where the peak inspiratory and expiratory flow rates are markedly reduced while the rest of the curve is relatively normal.

If an upper airway obstruction is suspected, fiberoptic bronchoscopy is the best way to confirm the diagnosis. Tomography can also be helpful, especially if it is considered too risky to introduce an instrument into the airway. Tracheostomy may be necessary depending on the degree and site of obstruction.

### Chronic Obstructive Airways Disease

Chronic Obstructive Airways Disease (COPD) generally is a mixture of chronic bronchitis and emphysema, although either condition may predominate. Chronic obstructive lung disease can usually be distinguished from bronchial asthma on the basis of the older age, long history of dyspnea, and the smoking habits of the patient. However, any patient presenting with a severe exacerbation of bronchial obstructive disease should be given the benefit of the doubt and treated vigorously to reverse any reversible component of the obstruction. Spriometry is a valuable aid to the diagnosis of chronic airways obstruction, but it must be stressed that patients who fail to respond to an inhaled bronchodilator may improve dramatically after an appropriate course of bronchodilator and corticosteroid therapy.

### Aspiration

Aspiration may provoke an exacerbation of bronchospasm or can masquerade as a refractory exacerbation. Many types of material can be aspirated into the lower respiratory tract, including small particles of food, foreign bodies, and varying quantities of gastric contents. Aspiration may occur when the severely dyspneic patient attempts to eat or drink. Nocturnal episodes of gastric acid aspiration may be a provoking factor in asthma. Finally, an aspirated foreign body may cause persistent wheezing and dyspnea suggestive of an asthmatic exacerbation.

## Thromboembolism

Thromboembolic disease can be very difficult to distinguish from severe asthma. There can be episodic cough, wheezing, dyspnea, chest tightness, hypoxemia, respiratory alkalosis, cor pulmonale, clear lung fields on chest x-ray, and apparent improvement after bronchodilators. The diagnosis should be considered if there is evidence of deep vein thrombosis or if their are risk factors such as venous stasis, hypercoagulability, or vessel wall injury. Generally the degree of dyspnea is greater and the degree of response to bronchodilators is less than in a typical asthma exacerbation. A perfusion lung scan, sometimes augmented with a ventilation scan, may help to establish the diagnosis, but the maldistribution of ventilation in the asthmatic may alter the perfusion scan and make scintiphotography difficult to interpret. At times a pulmonary arteriogram may be necessary if the suspicion of pulmonary embolism is sufficient to warrant the risk of the procedure.

## Pulmonary Venous Hypertension

The pulmonary venous pressure is elevated in a variety of cardiovascular disorders and may cause symptoms sufficiently resembling bronchospasm to warrant the description "cardiac asthma." Mitral stenosis is especially likely to present in this manner and can also cause expiratory flow obstruction on the spirogram. Pericardial constriction, left atrial myxoma, and left ventricular failure may cause wheezing and dyspnea similar to features of severe asthma.

## Hyperventilation Syndrome

Severe hyperventilation syndrome can appear quite alarming and may be associated with a severe respiratory alkalosis. The patient frequently complains of dyspnea and chest tightness and may have some wheezing. There is no expiratory flow obstruction on spirometry, and rebreathing expired air in a paper bag is sometimes dramatically beneficial. It should be remembered, however, that an asthmatic attack can provoke marked anxiety and hyperventilation in some individuals. Therefore, it is generally advisable to obtain a spirogram before dismissing the anxious breathless patient from the emergency room as a "hyperventilator."

## STATUS ASTHMATICUS

The term "status asthmaticus" connotes a severe potentially life-threatening process, unresponsive to the usual methods of treatment. It was used before the ready availability of arterial blood gases in the late 1960s and "usual" methods of treatment referred to aminophylline and epinephrine. The implication was that hospitalization and corticosteroids were needed. A better descriptive term would be "respiratory failure in the asthmatic," but "status asthmaticus" remains a useful expression if it connotes a respiratory emergency to the physician.

## HISTORY AND PHYSICAL EXAMINATION

Hospitalization is necessary when the patient falls into the category of status asthmaticus. In most instances, the asthmatic attack has been in progress for some days although there may have been periods of improvement. The patient is frequently on an erratic or inconsistent therapeutic program and may have visited an emergency room with temporary relief several times in the preceding week. An important clue is when the patient has slept little for one or two nights.

The patient is usually severely dyspneic, anxious, and diaphoretic. The degree of dyspnea can be defined by whether one's speech consists of sentences, phrases, words, or syllables. The respiratory rate may be misleading but suggests respiratory failure if the rate is over 35 per minute. Wheezing may be prominent or absent. A hyperinflated chest, prolonged expiration, prominent inspiratory recruitment of accessory muscles, and poor or absent breath sounds are important physical signs of the asthmatic in crisis. When there are visible contractions of the sternomastoids associated with elevation of the clavicles during inspiration, the $FEV_1$ is usually less than 1 liter.[5]

Pulsus paradoxus is also associated with severe expiratory obstruction and hyperinflation. When the respiratory variation of the systolic pressure is over 10 mm Hg, the $FEV_1$ is usually 1.25 liters or less.[6] There can be as much as 50 mm Hg of "paradox," which provides a quick method of assessing the severity of the obstruction and the response to treatment.

Tachycardia and hypertension are common. A heart rate of over 130 per minute is frequently associated with severe hypoxemia.

Restlessness, confusion, muscle twitching, hypotension, and disturbed consciousness are signs of established or impending respiratory failure and require immediate action.

### Laboratory Tests

Laboratory tests should be considered along with the previous clinical data. The arterial blood gas is an important method of monitoring the severe asthmatic. During a mild to moderate exacerbation, the $PaCO_2$ is typically reduced (35 or less) with or without a mild decrease in the oxygen tension. When severe hypoxemia develops ($PaO_2$ less than 50 mm Hg) and especially when the carbon dioxide tension rises to normal or even to 40 mm Hg or more, a sudden rapid deterioration may be imminent. The rising arterial carbon dioxide in the symptomatic asthmatic who is unresponsive to therapy suggests respiratory muscle fatigue and the need for mechanical ventilation.

Factors such as a pulse of over 120 per minute, respiratory rate of over 35 per minute, pulsus paradoxus of over 18 mm Hg, peak expiratory flow rate of less than 120 liters/minute, moderate to severe dyspnea, accessory muscle use, and wheezing have been used to develop a predictive index for relapse and need for hospitalization.[7] When each of these seven factors is given a score of 1, a total score over 4 is 95% accurate in predicting that the patient will relapse or need hospital care.

Several other laboratory studies should be obtained in the hospitalized asthmatic. A complete blood count can identify significant anemia, polycythemia, leukocytosis, and the presence of a left shift. The sputum Gram stain can help suggest a bacterial respiratory infection, but most respiratory infections in the asthmatic are viral.

Serum electrolytes, creatinine, blood sugar, and urinalysis should also be done. These are helpful in guiding fluid therapy and monitoring the impact of steroids.

A chest x-ray usually demonstrates hyperinflation or may show pneumomediastinum in the severe asthmatic. Occasionally a spontaneous pneumothorax may occur and will usually require immediate treatment. Evidence of pneumonia or atelectasis may also be seen.

The electrocardiogram usually shows sinus tachycardia. In the severe asthmatic, evidence of acute cor pulmonale may be seen. Arrythmias can be identified and treated if necessary.

## MANAGEMENT OF THE HOSPITALIZED ASTHMATIC

Bronchodilators, corticosteroids, hydration, and respiratory therapy are the major components of treating the hospitalized asthmatic. Endotracheal intubation and mechanical ventilation may become necessary, but if the patient can cooperate adequately, intubation can generally be avoided.

A frequent mistake in managing the acutely ill asthmatic is to delay therapy until the patient reaches the hospital room. A reversible situation may deteriorate while the patient lies on a stretcher awaiting transportation from the emergency room or the radiology department. Immediate steps such as starting an IV infusion and giving the loading dose of aminophylline and the first dose of corticosteroid should not be deferred until the administrative details of admission and the "stat" laboratory tests have been completed.

### Oxygen

The initial treatment would include supplemental oxygen, parenteral aminophylline, corticosteroids, and possibly a sympathomimetic agent. Concern about oxygen sensitivity should not prevent the use of adequate supplemental oxygen when hypoxemia is present. Severe hypoxemia is much more likely to cause serious damage than carbon dioxide retention. During the initial treatment of the severe asthmatic, we routinely use supplemental oxygen, even when the $PaO_2$ is in the 60–70 mm Hg range. We know that the arterial oxygen tension can vary considerably as a result of changes in position, intermittent plugging of airways from inspissated secretions, and the pulmonary vasodilating effect of many bronchodilating agents. A blood gas analysis provides information on gas exchange at one moment only, and in a life-threatening situation, it is safer to give oxygen and monitor gas exchange. The oxygen can be discontinued when saturations are adequate and the patients' condition has stabilized.

The most convenient way to administer oxygen is by nasal cannula. A flow rate of 2–4 liters/minute will provide an inspired concentration of approximately 30%–35%. Masks are rarely well tolerated by the severe asthmatic, but when it is desirable to maintain a constant inspired oxygen concentration, a venturi mask can be used. It delivers stable concentrations of 24%, 28%, 35% or 40% oxygen. A nonbreathing reservoir mask can supply the highest concentration of supplemental oxygen that can be achieved without endotracheal intubation (up to 70%). The reservoir device is seldom needed, except when there is an additional cause of hypoxemia and shunting such as pneumonia or heart failure. Careful blood gas monitoring is needed, no matter what is used to provide supplemental oxygen. It is desirable to keep the arterial $Po_2$ over 60–65 mm Hg and generally unnecessary to raise it above 80 mm Hg. If there is a significant degree of anemia less than 10 grams %, transfusion may be needed to increase oxygen delivery to tissues.

## Theophylline

A loading dose of aminophylline (5–6 mg/kg) should be given to adults not already on a theophylline preparation. If the theophylline level is subtherapeutic, a partial loading dose can be used. Patients already on therapeutic doses of theophylline should be given a maintenance dose of 0.2–0.5 mg/kg per hour. The lower dose is provided for the patient with known liver disease or heart failure. The maintenance dose can be readjusted in 12–24 hours after the theophylline level is obtained. A theophylline level of 10–15 $\mu$g/ml is optimal. The problems in determining the best maintenance dose of theophylline are discussed in Chapter 8.

## Corticosteroids

The prompt administration of systemic corticosteroids in an adequate dose is essential in treating the hospitalized asthmatic. Many asthma deaths could have been prevented if corticosteroids had been given in a more timely manner.[3] There is no scientific basis to recommend a specific dosage schedule, but our practice is to give large doses for at least 1–3 weeks.

Some patients with severe asthma have an increased metabolic clearance rate of cortisol. This is most likely the case in patients who have previously received corticosteroid therapy. An initial dose of 80–125 mg of methylprednisolone should be given as soon as the diagnosis of severe asthmatic relapse is made. There is little risk in giving a single dose of this size, and the avoidance of even a few hours of delay could be life-saving. The maintenance dose may range from 40 mg of methylprednisolone every 6 hours to 80 mg every 2–4 hours. A dose up to the equivalent of 4 g of hydrocortisone has been suggested.[8,9]

## Sympathomimetic Agents

Many chronic asthmatics have already received substantial doses of sympathomimetics, and it may not be desirable to use more during the initial phase of hospital treatment. The inhalational route provides bronchodilation with the least tendency for systemic adverse effects. Often the severe asthmatic has very irritable airways and will not tolerate any type of inhaled aerosol. In this situation sympathomimetics may be more effective when injected. Oral preparations are also useful, but many severe asthmatics may be in too much distress to take any medication orally. In general, there is more tachycardia, arrythmia, tremor, agitation, headache, and insomnia for a given bronchodilator response when sympathomimetics are taken orally or injected as compared to when they are inhaled. Additional details about the individual agents and their dose are provided in Chapter 9.

In a patient with severe bronchial obstruction the delivery of the bronchodilator from a metered-dose inhaler may be unreliable. Therefore, we prefer to give the nebulized solution over a 10–15-minute period. The occasional patient may benefit from an intermittent positive-pressure breathing (IPPB) device, perhaps because it stimulates a more effective cough. We use IPPB infrequently, but it seems to be valuable in a few patients. Once the patient can use the metered-dose inhaler adequately, we discontinue the nebulizer or IPPB device. The IPPB should not be used to treat progressive hypercapnia. In this situation, intubation and mechanical ventilation are urgently needed.

Bland aerosols tend to aggravate bronchospasm and so should not be used in the acute asthmatic unless they contain a bronchodilator or are given immediately after a bronchodilator treatment. Occasionally we may try a heated aerosol or ultrasonic nebulization to improve the delivery of water or saline to respiratory secretions. This may help to mobilize very tenacious secretions but may also stimulate severe bronchospasm. Mucolytic agents such as acetylcysteine are occasionally useful but may also greatly aggravate bronchospasm. Acetylcysteine may be more effective when administered directly through a fiberoptic bronchoscope into a regional bronchus obstructed with tenacious secretions that cannot be cleared by suction. Bronchoscopy in the severe asthmatic can be risky, and we reserve this for patients who cannot clear their secretions with the other respiratory therapy methods mentioned.

## Critical Care

It is often difficult to decide when conservative treatment has failed and whether the patient must be intubated. The need may be obvious if the patient is in profound distress on arrival at the hospital. The arterial blood gases are helpful, but there is no specific level of the carbon dioxide tension indicative of irreversible respiratory failure. Generally a patient on maximal treatment whose arterial $PCO_2$ rises into the normal range and above needs mechanical ventilation. Occasionally, a patient with an elevated $PCO_2$, usually one with chronic obstructive lung disease, may be able to cooperate with the respiratory therapy program and careful observation in the intensive care unit is sufficient. In the pure asthmatic, the combination of respiratory distress and rising arterial $PCO_2$ indicates that the patient is fatigued and that mechanical ventilation is necessary to prevent extreme respiratory failure from developing. Intubation may sometimes be necessary even with a decreased $PCO_2$. When it is obvious that the patient is tiring and has shown little response to aggressive treatment, it is better to intubate at this point rather than waiting for the inevitable deterioration in blood gas values.

To give some very rough guidelines, the patient who will need intubation will probably have one or more of the following reactions in spite of treatment: a vital capacity of less than 1 liter (15 ml/kg), an $FEV_1$ of less than 0.75 liters, a $PaCO_2$ above 40–45 mm Hg, a pulsus paradoxus over 20 mm Hg, a respiratory rate over 35 per minute, and difficulty in completing phrases or sentences because of dyspnea.

Once it is clear that intubation is needed, it should be performed without delay before the elective intubation turns into a cardiopulmonary resuscitation. Either the orotracheal or the nasotracheal route can be used, but nasotracheal intubation is usually more comfortable for the patient. The endotracheal tube should have a low-pressure high-volume balloon. The low-pressure balloon has been shown to reduce the complications of endotracheal tubes and allows at least 1–2 weeks of mechanical ventilation without tracheostomy.

Sedation is necessary after intubation and sometimes is needed during the procedure. Small frequent doses of IV morphine sulfate (1–5 mg/h) are usually quite effective. The cholinergic effects of morphine, theoretically undesirable, do not seem to be a problem in practice. The advantage of morphine over the nonnarcotic sedatives is that its effect can be reversed rapidly with naloxone. Diazepam (2–5 mg/every 1–2 hours) can also be used if necessary. When patients with severe asthma are not adequately controlled with morphine, a paralyzing agent such as pancuronium bromide may be needed. The recommended dose is 0.04–0.08 mg/kg. An initial dose of 5 mg followed by 3–5 mg every 3–4 hours is usually sufficient. Pancuronium is a nondepolarizing neuromuscular blocking agent that has no direct effect on cerebral function; therefore, a sedative should always be administered with it. The paralyzing agent should be discontinued as soon as possible. We prefer to allow the patient to wake up enough to communicate with us at least once or twice a day and to tell us, among other things, whether we have given enough sedative with the pancuronium.

A volume-cycled mechanical ventilator has the advantage of delivering a specific tidal volume. One can begin with a volume of 10–15 ml/kg, but this must be adjusted to avoid excessive peak inspiratory pressures. We try to keep peak airway pressure under 40–50 cm $H_2O$ to reduce the risk of barotrauma (pneumothorax, pneumomediastinum). Methods to keep the peak airway pressure low include using a paralyzing agent with a sedative, reducing the tidal volume, increasing the rate of mechanical ventilation, and reducing the inspiratory flow rate. Positive-end expiratory pressure (PEEP) is potentially hazardous in the severe asthmatic because of the risk of barotrauma and hypotension. It should be avoided except where there are unusual complications such as pulmonary edema.

A variety of other measures must be considered while an asthmatic is on mechanical ventilation. A nasogastric tube may be needed to decompress the stomach or to administer tube feedings. Antacids and sometimes cimetidine may be given to reduce the adverse effects of gastroesopageal reflux and to prevent stress ulcers. Minidose heparin (5000 units subcutaneously every 12 hours) reduces the risk of thromboembolism. Careful monitoring of fluid balance and hemodynamic status is also important.

Hypotension is sometimes a serious problem in the asthmatic on mechanical ventilation. The high intrathoracic pressure due to airways obstruction impairs venous return and loads the right ventricle. There is compression of the pulmonary capillary bed with each mechanical inflation of the lungs, and sedation may further depress the arterial pressure. Such patients need to be in positive fluid balance. They will often respond to a fluid challenge with saline, half-normal saline, or a colloid. If there is myocardial dysfunction or persistent hemodynamic instability, a bedside right heart catheterization can be used for measurement of the pulmonary capillary wedge pressure and cardiac output. Measurement of the mixed venous oxygen saturation is very helpful in assessing the tissue oxygen delivery.

Weaning the patient from the mechanical ventilator should begin when the broncho-spasm, retention of secretions, and unstable cardiovascular status have been sufficiently controlled. The severe asthmatic may require several days of mechanical ventilation before weaning can be started seriously. For weaning to be successful, any paralyzing agents must be discontinued and the dose of sedating agents reduced. Intermittent mandatory ventilation (IMV)[10] is a valuable technique for weaning in most patients. With IMV the patient is allowed to breathe independently but receives a fixed number of ventilator breaths each minute. This number is tapered gradually, with careful monitoring of the patient's clinical status and gas exchange. Specialized texts on critical care medicine should be consulted for more detailed information on the management of acute respiratory failure.

## CONCLUSION

Even with the best outpatient program, it is sometimes impossible to avoid episodes of severe bronchospasm that necessitate hospital care. More often, when an asthmatic must be hospitalized, the outpatient care has been deficient, usually because the patient has not been adequately educated about the need to adhere to the prescribed regimen and to seek help promptly when symptoms persist despite the usual therapeutic measures. On discharge from the hospital, the patient's program should be carefully reviewed and, when appropriate, there should be referral to others who can provide the education, psychological support, and additional medical interventions and monitoring that may help to avoid repeated hospitalizations.

## REFERENCES

1. Hudson L, Tyler M, Petty T: Hospitalization needs during an outpatient rehabilitation program for severe chronic airway obstruction. Chest 70:5, 1976
2. Lertzman M: Rehabilitation of patients with chronic obstructive pulmonary disease. Am Rev Respir Dis 114:1145, 1976
3. Ormerod LP, Stableforth DE: Asthma mortality in Birmingham 1975–7: 53 deaths. Br Med J 280:687, 1980
4. Ramsdell J, Nachtwey F, Moser K: Bronchial hyperreactivity in chronic obstructive bronchitis. Am Rev Respir Dis 126:829, 1982
5. McFadden E, Kiser R, DeGroot W: Acute bronchial asthma. New Engl J Med 288:221, 1973
6. Rebuck A, Pengelly L: Development of pulsus paradoxus in the presence of airways obstruction. New Engl J Med 288:66, 1973
7. Fischl M, Pitchenik A, Gardner L: An index predicting relapse and need for hospitalization in patients with acute bronchial asthma. New Engl J Med 305:783, 1981
8. Rebuck A, Read J: Assessment and management of severe asthma. Am J Med 51:788, 1971
9. Collins JV, Harris PWR, Clark TJH, Townsend J: Intravenous corticosteroids in treatment of acute bronchial asthma. Lancet 2:1047, 1970
10. Weisman J, Rinaldo J, Rogers R, Sanders M: Intermittent mandatory ventilation. Am Rev Respir Dis 127:641, 1983

Part 6

# Putting It All Together:
# Some Illustrative Cases

# Asthmatic Bronchitis in the Ambulatory Patient: Case Discussion

## A CASE HISTORY

I was recently consulted by a retired executive of a large international organization, aged 74, who had been troubled by allergic bronchitis for over 50 years. He experienced periods of cough and wheeze mainly at night, during damp weather, and when he had been in a dusty environment. He had been told that he was allergic to certain foods (peas, chocolate, tomatoes, and potatoes) and had avoided them for many years. During his early and middle adulthood he had only occasional attacks, but for the past 15 years he had never been entirely free of wheezing. Over the past 10 years he had been continuously on prednisone in a dose ranging from 5 mg daily to as much as 30 mg/day during exacerbations of his wheezing. He had been on various theophylline preparations that he tolerated poorly, complaining of nervousness and insomnia if he took his medication as prescribed. Four years earlier he had been given a beclomethasone inhaler with directions to take 2 puffs twice a day. However, he used it only when he felt he needed it and found it much less effective than the isoproterenol inhaler that he had used previously.

About 6 months earlier his symptoms had become more troublesome. He noticed that his sputum was thicker and that it took him longer to clear his chest before he could "get started" in the morning. On half a dozen occasions he had awakened during the night unable to breathe with a sensation of extreme tightness in his chest. He had gone twice to the emergency room of a hospital near his home where he improved after receiving some injected medication, and his dose of prednisone was increased temporarily. However, his symptoms returned fully within a few days after he resumed his usual schedule of medications.

He had no history of seasonal wheezing or rhinitis, but he was said to be allergic to a variety of pollens and dusts. There was no family background of asthma. He had never smoked. For a while he received "allergy shots," but they did not seem helpful and he stopped taking them after another physician told him that a person of his age "is never allergic."

### Comment

This story is typical of scores of patients we see every year at Scripps Clinic and, no doubt, is familiar to any allergist or chest physician working in a referral center. The patient had received most of the effective drugs available to treat asthma, but no attempt had been made to formulate a program to control his symptoms or to educate him about the purpose of his medications or when he should seek help from his physician. He was a very well educated and intelligent man in comfortable financial circumstances, but he had no idea that his asthma could be controlled on a much safer regimen than he had followed for over a decade.

Perhaps the worst flaw in his program was the long continued use of an inadequate dose of prednisone. Most patients who can be managed on less than 10 mg/day of prednisone are not truly steroid-dependent and can be successfully withdrawn from all glucosteroids or switched to topical treatment, provided that their bronchospasm is first cleared with an adequate period of intensive treatment. We see many patients who have been maintained for years on small doses of steroids, insufficient to do more than alleviate their symptoms but quite enough to expose them to long-term side effects. Often patients will taper the steroids prematurely, believing that they can reduce the harmful effects of the drug on their bodies by keeping the amount to a minimum. In fact, they only make themselves more dependent on the steroid treatment. Therefore, it is important when beginning a steroid "burst" to urge patients to stay with the full dose even when their symptoms clear, which they predictably will in a few days. Most patients do not appreciate the different magnitude of the risk associated with the short-term side effects such as sleeplessness, irritability, excessive appetite, and the very serious consequences of long-term treatment.

In our experinece the most common reason for poor results from beclomethasone is inadequate patient instruction. Most patients who are given this drug have used bronchodilator inhalers with immediate relief of their symptoms and find it hard to understand why the beclomethasone inhaler fails to give similar results. They must be told very emphatically that this is preventive therapy and that they must take it faithfully if they hope to be successful in tapering their doses of systemic steroid. There is no denying that it is a nuisance to use an inhaler three or four times a day, which makes it all the more important for the physician to explain clearly the purpose of the drug.

It has been only a decade or so since most people, patients and physicians alike, assumed that asthma was usually caused by allergies. When I first came to California in 1964 I was amazed to discover that many patients with typical emphysema believed that they had allergic asthma and were on stringent dietary restrictions in addition to regular desensitizing injections. Some even insisted that they had never been told that they should stop smoking. The pendulum has moved a long way in the other direction now, but we still see many patients being treated as allergic in the absence of any evidence that aeroallergens trigger their symptoms. As has been emphasized in previous chapters, the mere demonstration of specific reaginic antibodies does not imply that the patient has allergic asthma.

## THE FINDINGS

On the physical examination the patient was a youthful-appearing man with no abnormalities outside the chest. Forced expiration was moderately prolonged and there were diffuse medium to coarse expiratory wheezes.

The routine laboratory studies, including the chest x-ray, were unremarkable. Spirometry demonstrated evidence of moderate obstructive disease with an $FEV_1$ of 1.57 liters before and 1.80 liters after a bronchodilator aerosol was given.

# MANAGEMENT

There did not appear to be any question about the diagnosis, and so we proceeded immediately with more aggressive treatment, raising the prednisone dose to 40 mg daily. Mainly to see whether the patient would tolerate the drug, we began him on a long-acting theophylline preparation in a dose of only 100 mg twice daily, and to obtain a longer duration of action we prescribed a metaproterenol inhaler four times daily to substitute for the isoproterenol inhaler he had used irregularly.

Four days after his prednisone dose was increased, he reported by telephone that his nocturnal cough and wheeze were much better. He was troubled by some sleeplessness but otherwise tolerated the increased dose of prednisone well. We told him to increase the dose of theophylline to 200 mg twice a day and arranged for him to return for follow-up spirometry in 10 days.

Two weeks after beginning the prednisone "burst," the patient returned, delighted with the results of his treatment. His spirometric measurements had improved moderately, with the prebronchodilator $FEV_1$ rising from 1.57 liters to 2.07 liters and the postbronchodilator value from 1.80 to 2.51 liters. He had been troubled by heartburn, which had forced him to stop the prednisone altogether for 1 day, but the heartburn subsided after he began taking a liquid antacid preparation a couple of times daily. His serum theophylline level was 10 mg/1, which was considered high enough for a patient of this age, especially in one with gastrointestinal (GI) distress. He was especially pleased because he had made with impunity some cautious experiments in liberalizing his diet and was now indulging in the long-forgotten taste of potatoes every day.

In spite of his excellent subjective response, because he still showed a lot of reversible obstruction by spirometry, we decided to keep him on prednisone 30 mg for 10 more days and began him on beclomethasone 2 inhalations four times daily. After 10 days he was instructed to cut his dose of prednisone by 2.5 mg each day down to 15 mg daily and then by 2.5 mg every other day from the "off-day" dose until he reached 15 mg alternating with 5 mg. The 5-mg dose was selected as representing his previous "maintenance level." We planned to reduce his daily dose below that level only very slowly in order to avoid acute adrenal insufficiency.

He was seen again 7 weeks later after his initial evaluation, at which time his respiratory symptoms were entirely cleared and he reported no side effects from his medications, which he was taking as directed. He was advised to continue prednisone 15 mg every other day and to reduce the off-day dose by 0.5 mg weekly so that by about 3 months after he was first seen he would be on an alternate-day schedule of prednisone.

He followed these instructions, but over the next month while he was on a trip to Australia he became increasingly troubled by severe hip pain. He was seen by a rheumatologist who diagnosed aseptic necrosis of the femoral head, which was presumed to be due to his years of prednisone treatment. The drug was stopped over a few days without ill effect, and 4 months after we first saw him he reported that he had had no recurrence of wheezing after a month on only theophylline and inhaled beclomethasone.

## Comment

It is often difficult to persuade a patient who has been on prednisone for a long time and who is experiencing adverse effects that in order to lower the dose, it will first be necessary to increase it. This patient illustrates perfectly the problems that occur with "sending a boy to do a man's job" or using only enough prednisone to alleviate symptoms without completely clearing the bronchospasm. Many such patients, once they begin taking prednisone, experience what I like to call the "yo-yo syndrome," with symptoms flaring and remitting with repeated short courses and too-rapid tapers of the drug.

I almost always select prednisone because of its low cost, but prednisolone and methylprednisolone are acceptable alternatives. Long-acting oral glucocorticoids such as triamcinolone, dexamethesone, and betamethasone have no place in the treatments of asthma. I may start the ambulatory patient with an exacerbation of bronchospasm on divided doses of the steroid for 2–3 days but then almost always switch to giving the full dose with breakfast in order to minimize adrenal suppression.

Selecting the dose of prednisone is largely a matter of guesswork. I tend to use 25–60 mg/day depending on the age and sex of the patient, the current steroid dose, response to previous courses of prednisone, and my estimate of the likelihood of side effects. The common acute adverse effects tend to be reproduced with subsequent courses and most of them can be satisfactorily managed if they are anticipated. Sleeplessness, irritability, and mild emotional lability are common, but most patients will tolerate these symptoms if they are adequately warned to expect them. Usually it is not necessary to prescribe a sedative, but the patients and their spouses should be cautioned to report immediately if psychological responses are getting out of hand. Frank psychotic reactions occur now and again and may become full-blown over a couple of days if they are not treated promptly.

Although our gastroenterologist colleagues assure us that prednisone is not "ulcero-genic," a sizable fraction of our patients develop a very convincing facsimile of ulcer disease, complaining of hunger, epigastric distress, and heartburn while they are on these moderate doses of prednisone. We advise our patients to take the prednisone with food and to begin taking an antacid before each meal and at bedtime at the first hint of gastric symptoms. We do not hesitate to use cimetidine if antacid treatment does not promptly abolish the problem. With such precautions we do not recall ever having seen a patient develop a perforated ulcer or gastrointestinal bleeding while on a several weeks "burst" of prednisone.

In the early 1960s we and our patients often spent months "fighting the good fight" to avoid resorting to corticosteroid treatment, and when we finally took that dreaded step, it was usually with the expectation that patients would remain on steroids indefinitely and would probably develop the complications of treatment if they lived long enough. Now that we know better how to manage these potent agents, we are a lot less hesitant to initiate them, but it is very important at the outset to have a clearly formulated understanding of the goals of treatment and how we will respond to both success and failure.

It is essential to start with a large enough dose and to maintain it for long enough that when it is time to taper the bronchospasm will not promptly relapse. It seems more advisable to start with more than necessary and to reduce the dose slightly after a few days rather than to decide after a couple of weeks that the initial dose was too low. Problems with corticosteroid therapy are far more related to the duration of treatment than to the total quantity of medication given, and it is when the physician is half-hearted in the initial prescription that the planned "short burst" drags on for several months.

In many cases a week to 10 days on the high dose is probably sufficient to prepare the patient adequately for tapering, but for practical reasons we generally maintain the full dose for 2–3 weeks. Many of our patients live some distance away, and we rely on spirometry in addition to the subjective response to decide when the bronchospasm has cleared completely. A patient who is seen too early for a follow-up visit may be put to the inconvenience and expense of an extra trip, which, I believe, more than offsets the advantage of getting by with a few days less on prednisone.

Once it appears that a full response has been achieved, which may require an extra week or 2 on the high dose, our usual practice is to taper the dose rapidly, perhaps by 2.5–5 mg daily, down to 15 mg daily for men and 10 mg daily for women. These are generally regarded as the maximum "safe" doses for maintenance treatment, and tapering from this level can be accomplished more slowly if the patient proves difficult to wean. If the initial burst has been adequate, few patients will experience an exacerbation of their symptoms during this first phase of their withdrawal. This is an appropriate time to introduce inhaled beclomethasone because bronchial hyperreactivity should be at a minimum and patients are less likely to be troubled by cough when they use it. Inhaled beclomethasone should not be added to the program of an asthmatic who is not doing well on the existing program. Any recurrence of bronchospasm during the initial taper will indicate that the patient is problematic and you should be thinking about some of the special methods to deal with the steroid-dependent asthmatic at this stage rather than 9 months down the road after a compression fracture of the spine has developed.

The schedule of prednisone withdrawal from this point depends on the clinical situation. The patient with postinfectious bronchospasm without a history of perennial asthma can usually be tapered uneventfully over a few days. The chronic asthmatic who is not steroid-dependent can generally be tapered easily also, but should usually be maintained, for a few months at least, on inhaled beclomethasone. The patient with stable bronchospastic COPD who has responded well to a trial of moderate-dose prednisone should be tried on inhaled beclomethasone but generally will require a systemic steroid to maintain worthwhile improvement of his quality of life. Alternate-day prednisone therapy may be efficacious, but we do not hesitate to prescribe low-dose daily treatment if it is the only way to keep the patient reasonably comfortable. Sometimes these patients are exquisitely sensitive to small adjustments of their doses, getting along satisfactorily on 12 mg daily, for example, and relapsing on 11 mg. Therefore, it should be stressed to the patient that it is hopeless to try to reduce the dose in the face of increasing symptoms, as strong as the desire to discontinue prednisone entirely may be. Sometimes the refractory subject will not willingly accept this advice before experiencing a further exacerbation and repeating the prednisone burst.

It cannot be stressed enough that in order to use corticosteroid therapy successfully, the physician must be prepared to spend a lot of time explaining to patients and their families the purpose of the treatment and to frankly discuss the potential hazards and side effects at the outset. Patients will often receive much well-meaning advice from friends and relatives about the terrible things that may happen to them if they take the cortisone so recklessly prescribed by the "pill-happy doctor." Even the most compliant patients sometimes find it impossible to resist such propaganda and will show up in the emergency room after ill-advised attempts to accelerate their withdrawal schedule. Any physician who hopes to manage successfully a disease as chronic and devastating as asthma sometimes is must be prepared to work with the patients, recognizing that it may take some time to gain their confidence. Physicians who are personally offended if the patients choose to ignore their advice are likely to drive an asthmatic in need of competent help to an "alternative healer" less likely to provide it.

# Management of Severe Asthma in Relapse: Case Discussion

## A CASE HISTORY

J. W. is a 43-year-old businesswoman who had no respiratory symptoms during her childhood and early adult life. When she was 32 years old, she developed "sinus trouble" and at age 35 required a nasal polypectomy. When she was 32 she also experienced her first lower respiratory complaints. After a influenzalike illness beginning as a "head cold," she developed persistent cough, chest tightness, and wheezing. Since that time she has had chronic difficulties with rhinosinusitis and asthma, requiring maintenance treatment on inhaled beclomethasone, alternate-day prednisone, a long-acting theophylline, and inhaled metaproterenol.

She had smoked a pack of cigarettes a day for about 15 years but stopped at the time of her initial episode of flu-provoked asthma. She states that exercise, sudden changes in weather, and environmental irritants, especially smog, cause increased asthma problems. Her asthma also worsens with most upper respiratory infections.

J. W. was preparing for an important business lunch. She felt tense, was running a bit late, and developed a headache. At 10 A.M. she took two Excedrin (Bristol-Meyers Products, New York, NY) tablets. Following cocktails, she and her client sat down for lunch at approximately 1 P.M. Having never been to this restaurant before, she ordered something simple that she always enjoyed: broiled red snapper. Because this was a business lunch, she also ordered a bottle of white wine. Her luncheon choice came with a salad bar, and part of the way through her salad, she felt "uncomfortable". Thinking this was simply nerves, she drank some of her wine, but half-way through eating her entrée, she recognized that she was developing chest tightness and excused herself from the table. In the powder room she took 2 inhalations from her metaproterenol inhaler and returned to the table. Much to her surprise, the inhaler did not provide the normal relief from her asthma attack, and her wheeze steadily worsened. Her respiratory distress was now obvious and her client asked the maître d' to call an ambulance. When the paramedics arrived, they found her on the floor, barely conscious, but able to talk. She was cyanotic and in severe respiratory distress. They quickly ascertained that she was asthmatic and that she had been doing fine until shortly before they arrived. The paramedics administered oxygen and epinephrine and rushed her to the nearest emergency room. When she reached the hospital, although she was still in obvious respiratory distress with labored breathing, she was able to give an account of the entire episode.

When she was examined in the emergency room, she had a temperature of 98°F, a respiratory rate of 32, and her pulse was 100. Her blood pressure was 140/90 with 30 mm of Hg of pulsus paradoxus. She was visibly using her accessory muscles during respiration, and there were wheezes audible over the whole chest.

Analysis of the aerterial blood gases on 2 liters/min of oxygen by nasal cannula showed a $PaO_2$ of 60, a $PCO$ of 28, and a pH of 7.45. Spirometry showed that the $FEV_1$ was 1.34 liters with a predicted value of 3.24.

An additional 0.3 ml of subcutaneous epinephrine further relieved her symptoms, but after 15 minutes she was still wheezing. She was then given metaproterenol 0.2 ml in 2 ml of saline through a hand-held nebulizer, and after this treatment she was noted to be completely free of wheezing.

## COMMENT

When a patient appears in the office or the emergency room with a severe attack of bronchial asthma, it is important for the physician to have a well-formulated plan of action so that the initial evaluation can be performed and the effective treatment instituted with a minimum of delay. Our approach includes taking a pertinent history, performing a physical examination, and ordering diagnostic laboratory studies. A treatment program is worked out and its efficacy finally assessed so that a decision on postemergency management can be made.

## Assessment of the Patient

### *History*

An effective initial evaluation of a patient with severe asthma relapse must be rapid and specific. The key points to explore are the possible causes of the asthma relapse. This specifically refers to the provocative factors described in an earlier section of this text. Provoking factors most commonly responsible for an acute relapse of asthma include infection (most usually viral), exposure to irritants, IgE-mediated allergic asthma, food additives or preservatives, and use of aspirin or other medications likely to provoke bronchospasm, particularly beta-blockers (even timolol eyedrops [Timoptic Steril Ophthalmic Solution, Merck Sharp & Dohme, West Point, PA]).

The second important historical point is the duration of the asthma relapse. Is it something that just began so that the patient, although in acute distress, is well nourished, well hydrated, and rested, or has it continued for several days with the patient up at night and deprived of fluid and nourishment? The latter situation is obviously much more serious and hospitalization is more likely to be necessary. In J. W.'s case this was simple; the asthma relapse was abrupt.

One also must assess the medications that the patient is currently taking, not only asthma medications, but also over-the-counter preparations, looking particularly for possible aspirin and tartrazine reactions. It is important to determine the type of sympathomimetic inhaler and number of times per day *and night* the patient is using it. If the patient cannot remember or if you doubt the reliability of the answer, ask how many canisters of inhaler have been used since the attack began. The canisters contain about 200 inhalations and thus should last a month or so when used as directed. When an isoproterenol-containing inhaler has been overused, a syndrome may develop where each inhalation produces progressively weaker bronchodilation of shorter duration. It is also important to inquire about the use of theophylline and whether the preparation has been taken regularly and in an amount likely to provide a therapeutic blood level. One must also ask whether a glucocorticoid preparation is currently being taken in either systemic or topical form and in what dose. As noted in her history, J. W. was taking regular, alternate-day steroids, inhaled beclamethosone, and long-acting theophylline. She used these medications right up until the time of her acute asthma attack. In addition, she had used two inhalations of metaproterenol.

A final important point in the history is the course and treatment of prior asthma relapses. It should be ascertained whether the patient has been hospitalized because of severe asthma relapses in the past and if a corticosteroid was needed to control them. J. W. had never experienced an asthma attack like this before but prior upper respiratory infection-provoked relapses had required a "burst" of prednisone.

In assessing the duration of the relapse it is important to inquire as to whether the patient has had other emergency room or doctor's office visits for treatment of the present exacerbation. If so, it is much less likely that the asthma will respond to the usual emergency room measures without a period of hospitalization.

In the case outlined here, any number of possible provoking factors were active. J. W. recognized that irritants can increase bronchospasm, but she had handled smoky restaurants and bars before with her metaproterenol inhaler. She was nervous but never associated emotional factors with increased asthma activity. What about the aspirin? No! As it happened, the aspirin was, not responsible, either. Not because J. W. had taken aspirin before without adverse reactions. Aspirin sensitivity can develop at any time in about 10%–15% of the general asthmatic population. In patients like J. W. with underlying rhinosinusitis and nasal polyps (along with asthma, the "aspirin triad"), the incidence of aspirin sensitivity is as much as 30%–50%. J. W.'s physician should have advised her long ago to avoid aspirin and all cross-reacting nonsteroidal anti-inflammatory drugs. The reason that J. W.'s history does not suggest that the reaction was to the aspirin was the time element. She remembered taking aspirin at 10 A.M., and her reaction did not begin until about 1:30 or 2:00 p.m. Aspirin sensitivity, especially on an empty stomach, usually occurs within 1 hour, within 2 hours occasionally, and certainly never more than 3 hours after ingestion of the drug.

J. W.'s history suggested a reaction to metabisulfite, a widely used food freshener and preservative. She began to feel uncomfortable from the metabisulfite in her salad and unfortunately tried to calm her nerves with some white wine, which only contains more metabisulfite. J. W.'s history of severe smog sensitivity is consistent with what we have seen in sulfite-sensitive patients.

What about IgE mediated asthma from something she ate? First of all, isolated asthma without other symptoms of anaphylaxis would be a very unusual reaction to food only. Second, J. W. had had all these individual foods before without asthma; broiled red snapper was one of her favorite dishes. What was unusual at this new restaurant was the combination of salad bar plus the wine that she decided to add "for business purposes."*

## Physical Examination

The vital signs are a crucial part of the physical examination. One looks particularly for fever, tachycardia, and tachypnea. The respiratory variation of the blood pressure should be measured carefully in order to detect pulsus paradoxus, which is considered significant when the systolic pressure drops by 18–20 mm Hg or more with inspiration. One should auscultate the chest to look for wheezing, but it should be remembered that in some severe asthmatic attacks no wheezing may be heard because of the decreased intensity of the breath sounds. The chest movements should be inspected to evaluate the use of the accessory muscles of respiration. J. W.'s physical examination was as expected for someone with a severe acute asthma relapse.

## Laboratory Studies

The most important laboratory test in a severe asthma relapse is analysis of the arterial blood gases. Initially, in what has been called Stage I asthma the patient simply hyperventilates and the arterial blood carbon dioxide tension is reduced but hyperventilation compensates for the mild degree of ventilation–perfusion mismatch. Therefore, the oxygen tension level remains within normal limits. As the asthma progresses to Stage II the hyperventilation cannot maintain a normal $PaO_2$. The oxygen tension begins to drop, but the $PaCO_2$ remains low. In Stage III asthma the $CO_2$ tension begins to rise, but since the level was low in Stage I and II it appears normal in Stage III. It is essential for the physician to recognize that an asthmatic with a low $PaO_2$ and a normal $PaCO_2$ is not doing well and is likely to progress into respiratory failure as the $PaCO_2$ continues to rise. We consider asthma to be in Stage IV when the $PaO_2$ is less than 50 mm Hg and the $PaCO_2$ above 40.

Additional laboratory measurements include pulmonary function tests. The forced expiratory volume in 1 second ($FEV_1$) is probably the best predictor of the success of therapy and should be performed routinely. A complete blood count should be obtained. Anemia or polycythemia can complicate the acute asthma relapse, but the white blood cell count is of particular importance. There are a number of reasons why the white cell count will be elevated in asthma, including an acute phase reaction due to beta-adrenergic drugs or corticosteroids. Recent studies have shown that a total white count of 20,000 or more may be due to systemic corticosteroids alone, but that infection still is likely when there is a leftward shift of the differential count along with toxic granulation of the polymorphonuclear leukocytes. In addition, an increase in the absolute number of circulating eosinophils correlates roughly with the severity of the asthma.

A chest x-ray is rarely particularly helpful in bronchial asthma since the lungs

---

*For more information on aspirin-sensitive asthma, see Pleskow WW, Stevenson DD, Mathison DA, Simon RA, Schatz M & Zeiger RS: Aspirin desensitization in aspirin sensitive asthmatic patients, J Allergy Clin Immunol 69:11–19, 1982. For more information on sulfite sensitivity, see Stevenson DD & Simon RA: Sensitivity to Ingested Metabisulfite in Asthmatic Subjects, *J Allergy Clin Immunol* 68:26–32, 1981.

usually appear normal or simply hyperinflated, but it should be obtained in order to rule out pneumonia or a pneumothorax. Areas of atelectasis are commonly seen and should not be assumed to be infectious pneumonitis. J. W.'s arterial blood gases revealed Stage II asthma with hypoxia despite supplemental oxygen and a low $P_{CO_2}$. These are the expected findings in a young and basically healthy asthmatic in moderate to severe acute relapse. Despite the fact that J. W. was feeling better by the time she reached the emergency room, her $FEV_1$ still showed moderately severe obstruction. No other initial laboratory test would be necessary in this case.

## Treatment

### Measures to Avoid

In the treatment of the acute severe asthma relapse there are a number of commonly used therapeutic interventions that should be avoided as they are useless or positively deleterious. Inhaled corticosteroids and cromolyn are not useful in treating acute asthma and may actually provoke additional bronchospasm. Likewise, the use of a nonbronchodilator aerosol such as an ultrasonic mist in the acutely ill asthmatic may worsen the condition. Aerosols of acetylcysteine have also been reported to worsen bronchospasm. Intermittent positive-pressure breathing (IPPB) has not been shown to have any advantage over a hand-held nebulizer in treating acute asthma relapse and may in fact be deleterious. We avoid IPPB unless the patient's inspiratory effort is so feeble that the hand-held nebulizer cannot be used adequately. The high peak inspiratory pressure generated by IPPB could increase the risk of pneumothorax, and it has been suggested, although without convincing evidence, that mucus plugs may be wedged further into the bronchial tree. Patients with acute bronchospasm may be extremely anxious, but they should be given sedative medications only with extreme caution. Although the bronchospasm is inadequately controlled, sedatives are likely to worsen the respiratory failure. Once the bronchospasm has been effectively treated, the anxiety and sleeplessness commonly subside and no sedation is necessary. Therefore, think again if you are tempted to order a sedative for any asthmatic patient who the nurse reports as being unable to sleep.

There is little to be gained by giving sodium bicarbonate to correct acidosis since it has only a transient effect on the pH and it adds to the sodium load. Respiratory acidosis should be treated by improving the alveolar ventilation.

### Correct Therapy

Hypoxemia should be corrected by giving oxygen at a flow rate of 2–4 liters/min by a nasal cannula. The arterial blood gases should be measured again after 30–60 minutes and the oxygen flow rate adjusted according to the results. If the patient has chronic obstructive lung disease with $CO_2$ retention, the initial oxygen flow rate should be 1–2 liters/min.

If the patient has not had prior bronchodilator therapy; epinephrine at a dose of 0.3 ml of the 1:1000 dilution should be administered subcutaneously. This is especially useful in asthma associated with IgE-mediated disorders, particularly anaphylaxis, and also in younger individuals. Terbutaline at a dose of 0.25–0.5 ml subcutaneously is a satisfactory alternative. Either of these medications may be repeated at 15-minute intervals up to three times. If there has been no response after three doses, the patient can be considered in status asthmaticus.

A patient who has been given inhaled or oral beta-adrenergic agents without benefit should initially be treated as above with the addition of intravenous (IV) aminophylline. If the patient has not been treated before with theophylline or has not taken the prescribed medication regularly, a loading dose of 6 mg/kg of aminophylline should be given over 15–30 minutes followed by a maintenance dose of 0.2–0.9 mg/(kg h$^{-1}$) depending on the age and general condition of the patient (see Chapter 8, Table 8-1). If the patient has already been on a therapeutic dose of theophylline, an equivalent dose of aminophylline should be continued by a constant IV infusion, but it should be remembered that the metabolism of theophylline may be slowed during an acute illness. Metaproterenol solution by a hand-held nebulizer was used rather than additional subcutaneous adrenalin because J. W. was no longer in acute distress and would likely benefit from the decreased side effects and increased duration of action of the inhaled metaproterenol.

## Assessment of Response

A patient who responds rapidly to the measures described earlier can be discharged from the office or the emergency room within a few hours. If the attack is brief it can be assumed that the patient is not fatigued, especially if there are no other emergency room or physician office visits for this particular relapse. Studies have shown that 25% of the patients who are seen for their first visit for emergency treatment of asthma will ultimately need hospitalization. If a second visit is required, this figure increases to 83%. Presumably, by the time the patient has returned for treatment a second time, the spasm of the bronchial smooth muscle will no longer be simple. As the asthma continues, the airways become edematous, inflamed, and obstructed with mucus plugs.

Spirometery is a valuable aid in assessing the response to treatment. Favorable prognostic signs are a rise of 400 ml or more in the $FEV_1$ from the value obtained prior to therapy, or if $FEV_1$ is restored to 75% of the predicted value or 75% of the best value recorded before the relapse. A recent study used seven indices for assessing the response to therapy, giving each a value of 0 or 1. Hospitalization was necessary in 95% of patients with a score greater than 4. The indices included a pulse rate of greater than 120, respiratory rate greater than 30, pulsus paradoxus of greater than 18 mm Hg, a peak flow of less than 2 liters/sec, wheezing, moderate to severe dyspnea, and use of accessory muscles. No single parameter was independently useful to predict a successful outcome of treatment.[1]

When the patient is released from the emergency room, it is important to prescribe an ongoing asthma treatment program. All too often the patient is aggressively and successfully treated in the emergency room but is then sent home without adequate medication. Patients should be advised to avoid possible provocative factors, especially those likely to be responsible for the current relapse. Hydration should be maintained with an adequate fluid intake. One must optimize the bronchodilator program, adding inhalers and theophylline if indicated, and should consider using a new sympathomimetic agent or perhaps changing the dose or route of administration of the agent currently employed. One must also consider giving the patient a burst of a corticosteroid. This is more likely to be needed if the patient has required previous steroid bursts, especially if it is difficult to avoid the provocative factor responsible for the present relapse. Patients receiving long-term corticosteroid therapy should certainly be bursted following emergency room visits unless the attack is totally reversed or the provoking factor can be completely avoided.

If the patient has a poor response to treatment or is in status asthmaticus, as defined above, hospitalization is necessary. Treatment in the hospital includes adequate hydration. Although studies have not shown that giving fluids either parenterally or orally can influence the thinning or relative ease of production of mucus, asthma relapses of any duration with hyperventilation can be associated with significant dehydration, and in this state mucus can become more inspirated. The use of mucolytic agents is controversial and is discussed elsewhere in this volume. We regularly use inhalation therapy along with chest physical therapy, including percussion vibration and postural drainage to help to mobilize secretions. We generally prefer to administer a beta-sympathomimetic agent with a hand-held nebulizer rather than by IPPB for the reasons noted earlier. When the patient is able to tolerate it, ultrasonic nebulization can be considered, although there is some controversy as to whether the particles of moisture actually reach the small airways where they are needed. Aminophylline is continued IV at therapuetic doses. If the patient is hospitalized because of asthma, corticosteroids are essential. Doses should be adjusted according to the situation, but we usually begin with a bolus of 125 ml of methylprednisone and then give additional doses of 20–40 mg every 8–12 hours. We usually give two to three times the patient's maintenance dose if that patient is on long term corticosteroid therapy or has not responded to an outpatient burst. Antibiotics are not used routinely but may be started after sputum is obtained for culture if there is fever or expectoration of purulent-appearing material. Low-flow oxygen is continued and sedation avoided. Acute exacerbations of wheezing can be managed with subcutaneous epinephrine or terbutaline or with extra administrations of an inhaled sympathomimetic agent every 3–4 hours as necessary.

The program outlined here usually must be continued in the hospital for 5–10 days. When the clinical state improves and oral medications can be tolerated, the patient's program is converted to oral prednisone and a long-acting theophylline in a dose sufficient to provide a therapeutic blood level. One cost-effective way to evaluate the patient's progress is to collect all sputum in a plastic cup that is changed every 24 hours. The patient is ready for discharge when sputum production and mucus plugs diminish and when the spirogram returns close to its preexacerbation appearance. Studies have shown that even when symptoms disappear and the physical examination returns to normal, there is evidence of persistent airway dysfunction.

J. W. responded well to treatment (and time). The $FEV_1$ value rose to 2.60 and she felt "fine." At this point it was not clear whether her mild persistent airways obstruction was due to her years of smoking or if it represented some residual obstruction from her ongoing asthma. However, since the absolute value of her $FEV_1$ was a tremendous improvement over the initial reading, let alone what it must have been in the middle of the restaurant, and because we knew that the likely provoking factor was now completely out of her system, we discharged her from the emergency room to notify her regular physician about the incident and her suspected sulfite sensitivity. In addition, she was advised to continue her regular medication program and to avoid aspirin and nonsteroidal anti-inflammatory drugs.

## REFERENCE

1.  Fischi MA, Pitchenik A, Gardner LD: An index predicting relapse and need for hospitalization in patients with acute bronchial asthma. New Engl J Med 305:783–788, 1981

## SUGGESTED READINGS

Kelsen SG, Kelsen DD, Fleeger DF, et al: Emergency room assessment and treatment of patients with acute asthma. Am J Med 64:622–628, 1978

McFadden ER Jr, Kiser R, DeGroot WJ: Acute bronchial asthma: relation between clinical and physiologic manifestations. New Engl J Med 228:221–225, 1973

Shoenfeld Y, Gurewich Y, Gallan LA, et al: Prednisone-induced leukocytosis. Am J Med 71:773–778, 1981

ARTHUR DAWSON
RONALD A. SIMON

# 29

# Management of the Problem Patient:
# Case Discussion

## CASE HISTORY

In August 1981, we were asked to evaluate a 54-year-old housewife who had suffered from rheumatoid arthritis for over 25 years and from asthmatic bronchitis for 9 years. She exhibited the ravages of corticosteroid therapy that she had required continuously for 16 years.

She was well until, at the age of 33, she developed arthritis in the small joints of her hands and feet. Her arthritis became more troublesome 5 years later; but until 16 years previously she was successfully managed on gold injections, antimalarial therapy, and nonsteroidal anti-inflammatory agents. Since then she had required predisone in a dose that was never less than 5 mg daily and much of the time was higher.

Eight years ago she had her first attack of wheezing following an acute respiratory infection. She had smoked 20–30 cigarettes daily and continued to do so until a further episode of cough and wheeze 5 years previously. From that time she had experienced increasing respiratory difficulty with progressive exertional dyspnea punctuated by frequent exacerbations of bronchospasm. In the past 5 years her ill health was dominated by her asthmatic bronchitis, and although her arthritis remained troublesome, her steroid dosage was governed by the amount required to keep her bronchospasm at a tolerable level.

Eighteen months before we saw her she was hospitalized with a respiratory infection, requiring a further increase in her prednisone dose, and from that time had been progressively handicapped by persistent wheezing, severe muscle weakness, and depression. She had markedly cushingoid features and chronic steroid myopathy. During the last year she had suffered avascular necrosis of the right femoral head and of the right humerus, presumably also complications of her therapy.

Her physicians had made several unsuccessful attempts to maintain her on alternate-day steroid therapy and had also tried the troleandomycin-methylprednisolone combination discussed later which was abandoned because of gastrointestinal (GI) side effects.

We had planned to see her at Scripps Clinic for an elective outpatient evaluation, but a week before her scheduled visit her cough and wheeze had again worsened. She had increased her dose of methylprednisolone from 10 to 32 mg daily but was still in sufficient respiratory distress when she arrived that we decided to hospitalize her. In addition to the steroid, she was on theophylline, inhaled metaproterenol and beclomethasone, digoxin (for paroxysmal tachycardia), potassium chloride solution, amoxicillin, and occasionally flurazepam for sleeplessness.

She had a history of marked emotional lability and had been seeing a psychiatrist regularly. Much of her psychological distress she attributed to the effects of corticosteroid treatment that, she said, produced a "real Jekyll-and-Hyde personality change" when the dose had to be increased. The rest, quite plausibly, she related to her chronic debilitating diseases.

## Comment

Many of the patients we see with asthmatic bronchitis come to us almost "virgin." They may have obtained a bronchodilator from their physician or over the counter and perhaps will have been tried on one or more oral bronchodilator preparations, often fixed-ratio combinations, with no attempt to optimize the dose. Some have received no bronchodilator therapy whatever and have been treated only with numerous courses of ineffectual antibacterials, antitussives, and decongestants. With such patients the knowledgeable physician has a number of therapeutic options and treatment is often spectacularly effective.

Patients such as this present a very different problem. She was an educated, intelligent woman who had been in the hands of conscientious and well-qualified physicians. They had already tried all the standard methods of treatment in addition to using troleandomycin with methylprednisolone unsuccessfully. Her regimen had been worked out by trial and error over a number of years and appeared to be a reasonable one. There seemed to be little for us to do but to make minor adjustments of her program and to offer a second opinion in the hope that it would satisfy her that everything possible was being done.

## MANAGEMENT

In spite of the increase in her steroid dose her symptoms had progressed in the two days before her admission and so we treated her initially with a full program for an acute exacerbation of bronchospasm. She was given an initial dose of methylprednisolone 60 mg followed by 20 mg every 8 hours intravenously (IV). She was started on an aminophylline infusion, but we noted that she had a serum theophylline level of 20 mg/l when she arrived and so we lowered her dose somewhat, aiming to get her serum level in the area of 10–15 mg/l. Although her previous serum level was at the high end of the accepted therapeutic range, we suspected that mild theophylline toxicity might contribute to her insomnia and her paroxymsal tachycardia.

She seemed to have a poor response to metaproterenol when it was administered either by a metered-dose inhaler or as aerosolized solution, and so she was given a trial of a terbutaline aerosol that was prepared from the injectable solution. We also began her on a vigorous program of chest physical therapy, and four times daily she received chest percussion, vibration, and postural drainage. These measures proved very effective, and during her first 2 days in the hospital she coughed up a lot of tenacious secretions and her wheezing improved greatly. In the course of 5 days her forced expiratory volume (FEV) rose steadily from 1.14 to 1.94 liters and her cough, wheeze and sputum cleared completely.

Because of her arthritis we considered it important to rule out aspirin sensitivity. Once her bronchospasm had cleared, she was given an oral aspirin challenge test. On 2 successive days she received increasing doses of aspirin, initially 30 mg and finally 625 mg, which produced no demonstrable change in her forced expiratory flow. One of our rheumatologists saw her in consultation and concurred with the management she was receiving already, advising that she continue on gold injections, supplemented by aspirin if necessary.

She was also seen by one of our psychiatry group who noted that she had a long history of lability of mood with occasional paranoid ideation, generally when her corticosteroid dose was high. He also noted that a number of her relatives had been alcoholic and that the patient was in the habit of taking several drinks each evening although she had never considered herself a problem drinker. He recommended a trial of lithium therapy and issued a strong warning that she abstain from alcohol.

During her second week at Scripps we switched her back to oral medications and tapered her dose of methylprednisolone to 16, alternating with 4 mg daily. She then returned home and in the subsequent months was successfully managed on 16 mg every other day. With close supervision by her regular physician she was gradually able to resume some of the activities that she had been unable to perform for the previous 18 months. Although she continued to have many limitations, she felt that the trip to Scripps had been worthwhile, as much because it had helped her to come to terms with her illness as for the slight but significant improvement in her life-style she achieved in the succeeding 6 months.

## Comment

This story really has no punch line. We discuss this patient only to remind readers that some asthmatic patients do poorly in spite of the best care we can devise and that sometimes our efforts to treat them can be as devastating as the underlying disease. It is important to ensure that every therapeutic method has been explored and that experts are consulted when there is a question about any aspect of the patient's care. The woman in this case was evaluated by chest physicians, allergists, a psychiatrist, a rheumatologist, and an endocrinologist at our institution and had consulted physicians in several other specialties in her home community. It had not occurred to anybody before our psychiatrist saw her that lithium treatment might be beneficial; in retrospect, however, that was probably the most important contribution we made to her care.

There are a few general observations we can make about management of the problem asthmatic. First of all, a thorough search must be made to sort out all the possible provoking factors. Obviously in this patient, who had a fast resting heart rate and a history of sweats and paroxysmal tachycardia, hyperthyroidism had to be excluded. In any patient with a prior history of upper respiratory symptoms one needs to rule out occult sinusitis, the symptoms of which may be masked by steroids and antibiotics. If the patient has symptoms of rhinitis, controlling them may make the asthma more manageable since one of the major functions of the nose is to humidify and remove particles from the air before it reaches the lower respiratory tract. If the nasal passages are blocked and the patient breathes through the mouth, this conditioning function of the nose is lost.

Because the patient in this study had experienced severe side effects of corticosteroid therapy on the minimum dose required to control her wheezing, we considered trying her again on troleandomycin and methylprednisolone, but she did so well on standard treatment that we decided not to use this combination, since its results are difficult to predict.

Troleandomycin is a macrolide antibiotic related to erythromycin, which in combination with methylprednisolone has been shown to be useful in the treatment of some patients with severe corticosteroid-dependent asthma. We recently reported our experience with 16 patients who were on the maximum tolerated doses of bronchodilator and on long-term daily corticosteroid therapy.[1] In spite of being on a full therapeutic regimen, they still had persistent symptoms, abnormal pulmonary function tests, and repeated hospitalizations. Because troleandomycin decreases the clearance rate of theophylline, we first decreased the dose of theophylline by 25%–30%, depending on the serum level. Then the patients were switched from prednisone to methylprednisolone and troleandomycin. Further details of the protocol for using troleandomycin are contained in our report. All 16 patients experienced marked improvement in their asthma, and none were hospitalized during the follow-up period. The $FEV_1$ increased by an average of 39%. Before beginning troleandomycin, the patients were on an average steroid dose equivalent to 30 mg/day, and 14 of 16 patients required daily steroids. Following troleandomycin-methylprednisolone therapy the mean dose was reduced to 11 mg every other day, and 13 of 15 patients were able to tolerate alternate-day steroids.

Side effects were frequent but usually transient. Often there was an initial increase in the cushingoid appearance. Other adverse effects included GI upset, night sweats, and muscle weakness. Nine patients showed mild elevations in serum transaminase levels. Only one patient was forced to discontinue therapy because of intolerable GI upset. After the initial increase in side effects, most patients became distinctly less cushingoid than they had been prior to TAO-methylprednisolone once the dose was tapered and they were switched to alternate-day treatment. Additionally, we observed a return of baseline fasting cortisol levels in patients who had had no detectable adrenal function prior to beginning the program.

The mechanism by which the troleandomycin-methylprednisolone combination works is not known. The interaction with TAO seems to be specific for methylprednisolone because it is not seen with prednisone or prednisolone. Possibly the only effect of TAO is to increase the biologic half-life of methylprednisolone. This would explain why we initially see an increase in steroid side effects. However, it is difficult to see how mere prolongation of the effect of methylprednisolone could explain the later results. In the group of patients who responded, we achieved better control of the asthma on alternate-day steroid therapy while adrenal function improved and the side effects diminished. This suggests that troleandomycin has some more specific "steroid-sparing action" that affects the respiratory tract more than other target organs.

## REFERENCE

1. Zeiger RS, Schatz M, Sperling W, et al: Efficacy of troleandomycin in outpatients with severe corticosteroid dependent asthma. J Allergy Clin Immunol 66:438–446, 1980

# Index